Moving Forward

Life Changing Short Stories and Metaphors for Hypnosis, Hypnotherapy & NLP

by
John Smale

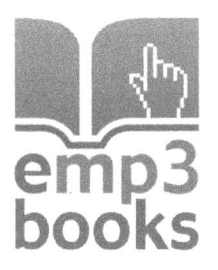

emp3 books

Published in August 2010 by emp3books Ltd
Kiln Workshops, Pilcot Road, Crookham Village,
Fleet, Hampshire, GU51 5RY, England

©John Smale 2010

The author asserts the moral right to be identified as the author of this work. All views are those of the author.

ISBN-13: 978-1-907140-19-8

All rights reserved. No part of this publication may be reproduced, stored in a retrieval system, or transmitted, in any form or by any means, electronic, mechanical, photocopying, recording or otherwise without the prior written consent of the author.

Limit of Liability/ Disclaimer of Warranty. Whilst the author and publisher have used their best efforts in preparing this book, they make no representation or warranties with respect to the accuracy or completeness of this book and specifically disclaim any warranties of completeness or saleability or fitness of purpose. The advice given in this book may not be suitable for your specific situation and is offered for guidance. The publisher is not offering professional services and you should consult a professional where appropriate. Neither the author nor the publisher shall be liable for any damages, including but not limited to special, incidental, consequential or any other damages.

www.emp3books.com

My thanks to the many people who have inspired the words that follow.

Other publications by the author include:

Mind Changing Short Stories and Metaphors
ISBN: 978-0-9550736-4-9

When used in NLP and hypnotherapy, metaphors have long given insights into the difficulties of people and have shown the ways in which we can escape or improve. Based on a huge amount of therapeutic work, these short stories, metaphors and interactive scripts can help you to bring about positive changes, eliminate negative thoughts and achieve your dreams.

Short Stories and Metaphors
ISBN: 978-0-9550736-3-2

When we look in a mirror we can see a reflection of how we are and how we want to be. The stories are based on the adverse effects that behaviours, attitudes and actions have had on the lives of others. They stem from the therapeutic experiences how people have exchanged their problems for happiness using short stories and metaphors and NLP.

The Secret Language of Hypnotherapy
ISBN: 978-0-9550736-2-5

Eliminating a few words from your thinking and your speech can change you, and others. Making a few subtle changes can persuade you, and others, to change minds. The secret and hidden language you need is contained in this book. You learn how to relax, hypnotise yourself and other people. You will discover how to overcome some of the major fears, phobias and personal problems of modern life.

Strictly for Therapists
ISBN-13: 978-0-9550736-9-4

Causes, Effects and Strategies for Effective Treatment with Hypnotherapy and NLP

More information from:
http://www.emp3books.com

CONTENTS

Introduction	1
The King and the Peasant Girl	3
The Snail and the Slug	8
The Sheepdog	10
West Meets East	14
The Village in India	17
An Awful Lot	23
Past, Present and Future	26
Substance and Abuse	28
The Drunken Truth	32
Growing Up, Growing Down	35
The Bullied Bully	39
Losing Your Temper	41
Change	45
The Saloon Car and The Sports Model	48
The Court Jester	52
Mythology and Fortune Telling	56
The Genie in the Bottle	59
The Puff-Adder	62
The Twelve Year Old Pilot	65
Elementary Truth	68
The Elements of Monkton Wyld	71
The Vanity of Power	72
Profit and Loss	75
Scar Tissue	80
Blackpool Rock	83
Previous Lives	85
Decompression	88
The Meat in the Pie	92
Living and Dying in the Past	94
Swimming with the Dolphins	99
Alienating the Aliens	100
The Root of all Evil?	103

Thou Shalt Not...but shhhh, I Shalt!	108
The Fat Mannequin	111
Felicity's Problem	115
What Is It?	120
Guilty or Not-Guilty?	122
Remote Control	124
The Confidence Trickster	128
Sperm	132
Air Mail	135
The Pearl in the Oyster	137
Memory	140
Ifs, Buts and Maybe's	142
Depression	143
Open Prison Walls	146
The Black Tunnel	147
Grains of Sand	149
Rolling Stones and Free Spirits	152
Moving Forward on The Life Train	154
Inner Wisdom	157
Dear Reader	158
Pinball	159

Introduction

The most perfect thing about humans is our lack of perfection.

Moving Forward is the positive outcome of that. We can realise that there is something better in the future. When we berate ourselves for not being perfect we wallow in failure.

When we see that the future can be better we thrive in the optimistic feeling that no matter what has befallen us there is always the opportunity for betterment rather than assuming that we have reached an end point.

As you read this book, either to yourself, to other people or to clients you will find answers and will be able to give insights into problems. This allows movement away from difficulties towards finding solutions and implementing them.

The decision to look at life from new perspectives gives the chance to earn your true value in the world and to profit from constructive change. Rather than being held back by old beliefs and attitudes, the reader moves into a new way of thinking, a new way of acting and a new way of life.

Taking and acting on decisions is paramount to success. By moving forward now, you invest in a brighter future.

And a darker view.

Some of the metaphors are dark. They tell tales of abuse and the nasty nature that some people have. However, the darkest hour is just before dawn. The darker stories offer hope to those readers who can identify with them. The outcome is about moving away from the past into a brighter future. Just because bad things have happened before there is no need to assume that the victim is cursed with a life that repeats the hurt.

The end of every ancient story is justice for the wronged and the chastisement of the perpetrator. So it is with these tales and so it should be.

These stories and metaphors help the readers to climb out of the mud that holds them back and delivers them into a place where they can be fulfilled and happy.

And a view in verse

A few metaphors are presented in verse form as they use images and analogies to create an atmosphere. Some are about being stuck in seemingly immovable situations and show a way forward. They are dotted through the book to give elements of change.

The King and the Peasant Girl

The King was a sad old fool. He thought that he could get anything that he wanted because he was a King.

The Queen did as much as she could to keep him happy. She would kiss him, she would cuddle him. She would do whatever the King wanted.

One day the King was riding around his Kingdom on his large white horse. It had to be the largest horse in the land because he felt so very important. In a small village he spotted a young girl going about her business of tending to the cows. The King stopped his horse and dismounted. He walked over to the girl and asked her if she knew who he was. Of course she did. There were pictures and statues all over the place. His ego was as large as his Empire.

The King was very taken by this young lady and his desires grew beyond those that he felt for his wife and other young girls he had met. After all, this one was fresh and innocent, she was very pretty and, after all, he was the King.

He needed a plan. He told the girl she was a very special person and she could help him to rule the country. He told her that she would have to keep her role secret as there were very many spies around. He arranged to meet her the next day in their secret place.

Day after day for a few weeks the King would arrive at the corner of the field where he had first seen her. He brought her presents of precious jewels that were really glass marbles. He would give her sweets from the kitchen in the palace.

Then he said that because he trusted her so much he would make her an honorary Princess.

To do this, and because it was a secret, he would anoint her in a private place. She laughed and said that they were in a private place already. He ran his hand along her leg and touched her on a part of her body that nobody had ever touched before. She was, at once, shocked and a little pleasured by this. After all the King had told her she was special.

She knew that what had happened was wrong but she was confused by the sincerity of the King. He would not tell her lies or do anything that was inappropriate.

The next day it happened again and she resisted. The King told her that she was the one who had wanted to be a Princess and that she had encouraged the King to touch her on that part of her body. The King told her that if she informed anybody about what had happened then he would have her head cut off, and to her, more frightening was that he would cut off the heads of anybody she told,. That included her parents.

The girl had to protect her parents and she allowed the

King to carry on with the touching. She even complied when he told her that she should touch him. She said that he knew what had happened and told him to stop. She asked him if he ever told anybody if his head would be cut off as well. He laughed.

The King was all powerful. Nobody questioned his disappearances every day. The girl became worried about what was happening but was convinced that it had been her fault.

After all, the King had told her so.

One day the King went even further with the girl. He told her that what happened was part of her initiation into the world of royalty. Her tears and her pain were compared to the lonely all-night vigils of knights before they were dubbed with a sword.

There is no need to give more details but the upshot was that after that happened a few more times the King was impressed by another young girl who he had seen whilst riding to meet with the victim of our story who never saw the King again.

This ten year old girl grew into womanhood with the belief that she was wicked and evil. She allowed some of the men in the village to use her because they would say nice things to her to get their way but they would always run away afterwards, just like the King had done.

He had convinced that she had no value and that she

was unwanted for anything apart from satisfying the wants of men.

She left her village and walked for days until she crossed the border into another Kingdom. There she decided that she would start a new life.

One day in this new place a handsome young man saw her. He dismounted from his horse and started an open courtship. He was gallant and charming. He was interested in her as a person rather than just a as a body that could be used for his pleasure.

One day he told her that would be unable to see her for a while because he had to lead soldiers into a war with another country. She believed that, like all the others, he wanted to be rid of her.

He was going to the country that she had come from to depose the wicked King who had robbed the people with high taxation to pay for his openly debauched way of life. The Queen had left him and now lived in exile.

The girl's parents still lived in the village where she had been born. She needed to warn them about the war. She walked back along the route she had followed a few years before. She followed the trail of battles until she arrived at her home.

The news was that the King had been beaten and was about to be executed. His fat body was kneeling at a chopping block, the axe high in the air. The girl walked over and told everybody that this was the man who had abused her.

Other girls did the same.

The head that was lost was not the girl's, not those of her parents, not those of the other girls.

A huge cheer went into the air as the axe fell.

The girl felt a tap on her shoulder. Her young man was standing beside her dressed in the finest armour. He told her that he was a real Prince and asked her to marry him. She told him that could not happen because she was evil and that she had seduced the King.

The Prince laughed and told her that he had never met a young girl who was so wily that she could do such a thing but that he had met many men who used cunning and guile to abuse the innocent. The real villain had lost his head that day and the real heroine also lost her head, but this was to a Prince.

Very often victims of abuse are made to believe that they were in some way responsible for what happened. This is a fallacy. Abusers are adept at planning their acts and at using the innocence of youth to convince the victim of culpability. They work like military tacticians in getting what they want and never worry about the damage that they cause to their victims. If you are a victim, or if you know victims, then you should realise that abuse attacks the mind as well as the body. The innocent are always innocent and the perpetrators are always guilty.

The Snail and the Slug

The slug and the snail were the best buddies than any gastropod could wish to have.

They spent hours munching away at plants and decaying matter. The one problem that they had was that the slug was envious of the snail's shell and wondered why he was born deficient of protection. The lack of shell made the slug less attractive to all the other creatures in the garden. Although a lot of people could cope with snails, nobody liked slugs.

A French garden is a joy for wildlife. Jean-Claude, who had the garden these friends lived in, grew a huge variety of crops. Asparagus, lettuces cabbages and, of course, garlic, along with the many other tasty plants.

One day Jean-Claude was harvesting his bounty when he decided to collect the snails that were eating his vegetables. He avoided the slug, too ugly, too slimy, and very revolting.

The slug was intrigued by the collection of his neighbours. Perhaps they were being invited to a feast.

They were, as it happened.

The slug moved, at a snail's pace to the wall of the kitchen. It climbed the wall slowly until it reached the window. Adjusting its eye stalks to obtain a good view he saw the snails, one by one, being dropped into a cooking pot. He saw his friend being picked up. Just as he was being dropped into the pot he saw the snail, his best friend, look at him with tears in his eyes. He was envious of the slug's lack of a shell, a portable house.

The slug dropped to the ground and made its way to the bottom of the garden.

The following day Jean-Claude emptied his recyclable rubbish onto the compost heap. Usually a source of good waste for the slug, this new arrival contained shells. As he made his way towards them he saw the empty shell that had belonged to his best buddy.

Rather than climbing into it the slug thanked its lucky stars that it had never had a shell. He had avoided being caught, being cooked and being eaten with garlic butter.

Then the frog snapped him up. The time for the end of a great friendship had come for both of them for the time being. When the frog was caught and its legs eaten, the essence of the two best buddies met each other again in Jean-Claude's stomach.

We have to be grateful for what we have rather than be unhappy at what we do not have. When we envy others we should use our desires to motivate us to do more to move forward in our lives to achieve what we want. Envying others never gets for us what they might have. Only our own efforts will achieve our goals.

The Sheepdog

The shepherd was feeling nervous, he was feeling anxious. He worried about the cost of food for his sheep; he worried about the market values of meat. He worried about paying his tax bill. In short, he worried about so much; nearly everything.

He had a sheepdog called Jackson. This dog was his everything. He was a pet when company was needed; a tool with the sheep in the field and a prized possession at the sheepdog trials. Jackson was the love of this man's life. The shepherd would dream about the two of them running through fields, catching balls, playing in the surf of the ocean and frightening rustlers away.

One night the shepherd had a different dream. He and Jackson were surrounded by evil sheep in a gigantic meadow.

These sheep were different. They had razor sharp horns, the teeth of crocodiles, the claws of eagles. They were evil predators.

In his dream, the shepherd and Jackson had the job of rounding them up and trapping them in pens. The shepherd was scared and if anyone had witnessed this dream they would have heard him screaming in his sleep. Jackson was alarmed as he lay by his master's bed.

These monstrous sheep transformed in the dream.

One became a huge ravenous dragon that poured fire onto the small piles of bank notes that represented the shepherd's meagre savings. The ash blew away in the breeze. Another sheep became a disease that kills ordinary sheep. Another was jumping heavily so that the ground cracked as if an earthquake were happening. His farmhouse disappeared into the ground.

With every new transformation the threat and malevolence increased. The shepherd knew that he was dreaming, having a nightmare, but was unable to reach the safety of being awake. He was trapped with his foes in a land over which he had no control.

Jackson set about his business. With deft ability he chased the monsters, he herded them and then, snapping at their ankles above the claws, he herded them into the pens. When they were in there they seemed to revert to normal and docile sheep. No threat, no wickedness.

Yet there were many of them and it seemed to go on for hours. The shepherd helped Jackson by shaking his stick and shouting at the brutes.

At last they were all under control. They were all set in the pens where they all became as they should have been.

Then a ram hurtled into the field. He ran to the

shepherd, its head lowered, ready for the butt that would end the shepherd's life. Time slowed for the shepherd and he saw that all the sheep represented his anxieties and worries. If he rounded up those fears, if he controlled them then he would gain his life back. He would start to win.

In this dream he saw that he needed to take control of his anxieties and fears. He had to stop them from worrying him, from attacking his quality of life. In those few moments before he would be tossed into the air like a rag doll, he wished that he could have another chance to take control of his life.

The ram was closer, its apparent slow motion lethargy never disguising the bulk and ferocity of the creature. This had the appearance of the greatest unease that could be felt. It made the shepherd sweat. His heart-rate reached an all-time high, his breathing was fast and rapid. The ram's name was Panic. The shepherd was under attack.

As its large head smashed into the shepherd's forehead, the slow motion made it feel like a soft caress. He opened his eyes to see Jackson gently licking his face.

The dream, the nightmare, had ended but his new life and his hopes, like the sheep, had transformed. But this change was benevolent rather than evil.

He got out of bed. The lamb chops sizzled on the stove. He and Jackson had the best breakfast ever on this new morning of a new life.

"We are having pan-fried Panic for breakfast, Jackson. See how he likes it when he is put in his rightful place."

The shepherd had discovered through his dream that when anxieties are sorted, controlled and penned they become passive things. It is only when they run around and threaten that they become dangerous.

Taking control unto himself was the answer. When he was controlled by everything outside himself he was nothing more than a puppet dancing to a tune not of his choosing.

Being one of the crowd, following like the sheep in our fields only ends up with us being in the slaughterhouse of our aspirations for life. Like Jackson, be a free spirit and herd the causes of your worries into a place from where they cannot escape.

West Meets East

Pictures from the air do not seem to tell the whole truth. The first thing visible from the 'plane was the most magnificent sunrise graduating from blackness, through stripes of red to orange, yellow, green and blue. I expected Delhi to match those bright colours but instead it was covered in a blanket of fog. Fog and a few matching airport concrete buildings were all I saw of Delhi while sitting on the aircraft, delayed, waiting for take-off to Bombay. "Delayed for the movements of a VIP" was the pilot's explanation. I said to my neighbour, "He's a long time in the toilet." My comment had no response other than a raised eyebrow.

The first view of Bombay suggested a collection of abject misery. Small and numerous shacks lined the approach to the airport. The 'plane seemed to almost clip some of them.

After landing and the various lengthy immigration formalities I took the free bus to the domestic terminal, the wrong one as it turned out! After ridding myself of numerous airport hotel touts I took another bus to the correct terminal.

From this bus I saw the shacks at close quarters, some housing people, one housing about eight buffalo. These sheds by Western standards were horrible (although I have seen similar on the outskirts of Paris). The inhabitants, however, looked relaxed, almost like tourists on holiday in the Mediterranean resorts, keeping out of the sun, smoking, piddling. They were happy with this way of life. I suppose they were in a community where all were equal, no snobbery, just sharing life.

Every so often the bus stopped and some of these people caught sight of my white face. The look they gave was one, not of jealousy as my Western arrogance might suppose, but contempt, a withering look that made me feel out of place, so alien.

I wondered if this was the look that some of my ancestors gave and some of my countrymen give to immigrants, the "you're not welcome here because you are visibly different" look. These people do not have to worry about foreign investments or being servile in the tourist industry. They can express what they really feel.

Flew to Bangalore.

The hotel is fine. Air-conditioned and mosquito proof.

Dinner quite magnificent. I had a mixed platter of chicken drumsticks, pink even though well cooked, like chicken was in my childhood, marinated chicken, Tandoori chicken, paneer and wonderful kebabs. Also some vegetable pulau rice. So much that, hungry as I was, I left some rice and a drumstick!

Eating is strange. Here I am a well fed Westerner eating thin animals. I have visions of the thin men walking barefoot along the road, covered only in sackcloth. I left so much food because the portions are so large. What I left would feed so many. The poor animals I see in the fields, so thin and ragged are used to feed fat people to make them even fatter. No wonder so many people here are vegetarian!

Back in Bombay I was taken to the "Gateway to India" which is so unimpressive that it should really be called the hole in the fence. Saw a real snake charmer plus his live cobra. He crept up behind me when I was talking and when I turned to see who was making the music I saw the poor snake, thin and small and black.

Made me jump at first but I actually felt sorry for a wild, powerful and fearsome thing being made to play to a crowd for rupees. Apparently they are swung by the tail when first caught so that any venom is disgorged by fear and centrifugal force. Their fangs are then removed by pliers together with their poison glands.

Snake charming is now illegal in India and the charmers are fined and the snakes taken to local zoos.

This is taken from the author's diary after going to India for a work project. This meant that rather than being a tourist I was helped and guided by work colleagues. The diary is included because it gives a sense of contrast in terms of lifestyle and value. This was written in 1994 so it relates to India at the start of the huge changes that have added Western styles to the country.

PS The man in next story is NOT the author!

The Village in India

The well-off businessman was being driven through a remote part of India. The monkeys were hopping from branch to branch in the trees, the birds were circling overhead. The scene was idyllic.

The car entered a small village. The man saw three women with a cow. One woman held the cow with a loose rope around its neck. The second woman was doing the job of extracting milk from the teats. The third, a very pretty girl, was feeding the cow with grass. All four looked content and happy.

The businessman could always get what he wanted and the girl was on his list of required acquisitions.

Further into the village the huts stood in casual rows. Children played. Old men sat with their friends to talk about whatever. The older women were preparing food for their families.

This was the Garden of Eden. People were without riches that they could spend but they had an abundance of the things that money cannot buy.

The businessman did not see it that way. He was an acquisitive man and his idea of contentment was to have things.

Upon returning to his hotel he made phone calls and

within days a huge television set and satellite aerial were delivered to the village. A generator, complete with fuel, was set up to power the TV.

Soon after, he was driven to the village where everybody was grateful to him for what he had done. He asked to see the girl who had been milking the cow on his first day there.

She walked to him, bowed and smiled coyly before politely walking away so as not to embarrass him. The businessman was happy. He had gone some way to appeasing his conscience for being so rich. After all, he persuaded himself, after his life of deals that left some people poor but his company successful he wanted to give something back. He wanted the girl to be so impressed that she would want to visit him on his own territory.

A month later he was driven back to the village expecting the inhabitants to be grateful to him for his generosity. So grateful, indeed, that they would offer him the gift of the girl in return.

He found chaos, he found ruin and he found unhappy people. He asked his driver to translate the comments of these villagers.

"They say that they need cars. They say they need a swimming pool. The girls want make-up and fashionable clothes. The men want designer shirts and underwear. They say that the TV has shown them what is in the world that they cannot have. They want you to buy those things for them."

The businessman was wise, to an extent. He told the people, through the interpreter, that he would fix things. He saw the girl he liked and she smiled at him again but he saw that she was disguising a sneer.

He was driven back to his hotel and made phone calls.

Within days the television, the aerial and the generator were removed.

He told his driver, sarcastically, that these people could now return to the happy way of life that they had previously.

After another month he again returned to the village. He still craved the girl.

There had been an even greater change in the small community. The inhabitants were even unhappier. They had been shown a way of life that had been unknown. Then they had been left to struggle along.

So the younger and fitter young people left the village and walked to the towns to look for the work they needed in order to provide all the things that they had been deprived of. They worked like slaves for meagre wages that barely kept them in food.

Nothing could ever bring back their simple sense of satisfaction with life. The businessman had thrown them out of this Paradise and had closed the door behind him.

Having been thrown out of Heaven they now knew the Hell of the factories owned by the well-off businessman.

He told very few people, if any, that his dream all along, had been to impress and seduce the pretty girl who was feeding the cow in the village when he first drove through.

She, at first loved the idea of the mogul and then disliked him for what he had done. He had given his game away when he had slipped her a note, in English, saying that he could make her rich beyond her dreams if she would warm his bed.

On that last visit she had asked the chauffer to translate the note. She did not speak English. She had then asked the chauffeur where the rich man lived. She was told the name of the hotel.

She walked the long distance to the hotel, asked for the man's room number. She climbed the stairs, moved along the corridor and found the door. She dropped an envelope onto the carpet, covered it with her best sari and knocked.

When he answered the door he was excited, he was ecstatic.

She entered the room and stood still, looking at his expectant face. She slowly slipped out of her sari and stood naked in front of him. He could see her slim waist, pert breasts and the dark triangle of curly hair that pointed at his desired target.

He discarded his clothes across the room. As he moved towards her she held her hand up to stop him, as if teasing.

She backed up to the door, grabbed the handle and left after wrapping her waiting sari around her. She ran as fast as she could. As he tried to run after her he realised that he was naked. The door slammed shut behind him. He was trapped by circumstance.

He saw the letter on the floor. He grabbed it to cover his modesty as he called for help.

After he had been let back into his room he became very angry but he opened and tried to read the letter.

After he had dressed he took the letter to reception for translation.

It said:

"Before you saw me you didn't want me because you had no idea that I existed. When you saw me you wanted my body, not me. After you saw my naked body you craved for it.

When I had left your room then you knew what you wanted. Then you knew that you could never have it.

Your gift of the television did that to every single villager. You ruined lives not out of a cruel mistake but because you wanted to buy minds and bodies.

By the way, never visit the village again. I will not be there. I am going to live with my relatives far away.

Goodbye, sad man.

Rather than getting angry he was saddened. The spirit, mind and body of this girl made her even more desirable. This became a greater loss for him than it had been before. He knew how the villagers must have felt.

Afterwards, despite lavishing the villagers with gifts that satisfied rather than frustrated, he was never forgiven.

Yet, the greatest punishment for him was that he never saw the girl again apart from in his mind and imagination.

When we live in a good place we can be seduced by the idea of the unattainable. The striving to find it can destroy the very fabric of happiness. Sometime things are best left as they are.

Buying hearts and minds will only give short term results. After the cynical motivation has been exposed then the real intention becomes apparent.

An Awful Lot

Gordon had an average sort of life. He had a wife, an average car, an average house and average expectations from his existence.

His dream was to win the lottery. When asked how much he would like to win he would just say, "An awful lot of money".

He bought his tickets every week using his usual numbers but one day, because it was a rollover jackpot, he splashed out on a lucky dip ticket.

To put it briefly, he won an awful lot of money.

He rushed out and bought a big house complete with a swimming pool. He bought himself a fast car that he would impress everybody with. It was his big win so he decided to keep the money to himself. His wife, he perceived was old, even though she was five years his junior so he visited bars and clubs and found himself a girlfriend who was half his age. She was very well qualified in spending money and she was very demanding. She wanted diamonds and gold. She needed the finest food from the finest restaurants and she demanded a fee whenever they made love.

He had an awful lot of money and it was all worthwhile, for him, anyway. He could afford great lawyers and he removed his wife from his life at a reasonable cost.

He found his friends from the past were distancing themselves from him, probably because they were jealous of his wealth, he reckoned. He could afford to buy new ones anyway.

He became bored with his girlfriend and he invested in new ones, even younger and prettier.

One of them, Mona, was an investment analyst and gave him tips on how to spend his money to get the best return.

After a few wonderful deals that she had told him about he was very happy to invest all his savings, all his assets and all his faith in the deal of deals.

Mona told him she needed to fly to South America to ensure the deal was fully set. He waved her off from the airport, returned to his big house, took a swim in his warm swimming pool and relaxed with a huge cigar.

He heard nothing from Mona, no phone calls, no texts, and no mail. He was worried about her safety.

The security gates sounded the arrival of somebody.

He looked at the CCTV monitor and saw two men in suits standing there. He worried that some tragedy had befallen the girl of his dreams. He let them in.

The bailiffs did not take too long to eject the man from his house, seize the keys to his car and leave him locked out. He was penniless, homeless and loveless.

He telephoned his ex wife and asked for help. She was delighted to hear from her ex-husband and offered to pay for him to "go to Hell", as she put it.

"I need you back, I love you." He pleaded. She laughed. "I will do one thing for you. I will give you enough money to buy one more lottery ticket. You always wanted an awful lot of money. That is what you got. The money you won gave you an awful life. I will give you the chance to win more money that will be even more awful for you to have."

She hung up and got on with her less than average life.

She had invested the little money she had been given by her husband's lawyers and had been handsomely rewarded. She had a nice lot of money, now.

She smiled at her new partner and laughed loudly for a good few minutes before starting work again in the animal shelter that she had bought.

Money that is used selfishly can turn out to be a poisoned chalice. If the universe is kind enough to share its wealth with somebody then the recipient should be kind enough to use the good luck to benefit the World and it occupants. Money is very rarely free.

Past, Present and Future

"I wish that I had a time machine" He thought.

"If I had one then I could travel into the future and see my destiny. I could even make it happen because I could know the way the world will be. I could investigate the technology and bring it back so that I could invent it and make loads of money.

"If I had a time machine I could travel back to my past. I could erase the mistakes that I made and build a better life for myself."

The thought came that a lot of the wish was to change things that should have never have happened and to rewrite the actions that had led to a place less comfortable than is wanted.

He continued his thoughts. "My future desires are the theft of the ideas and work of other people. It would be too easy to take the developments yet to come. If Hitler had a time machine then he might, no, certainly would have, developed the nuclear bomb and used it. We would not be here. I could not have gone back in time and shot him because I would not be here, now.

"If I had a time machine and could go back into the past then I could have stopped being a jealous man. I could have prevented the things that I can see were wrong and damaging in hindsight. I could have worked harder, I could have planned a better life. If only..."

What was missing from his thoughts was the idea that we make our futures by what we do in the present. We need to think about consequences. We need to control how we react and how we relate to other people, the creatures of our planet and the world itself.

We have a time machine within us but one that can change the future by considering the present.

If we had a time machine in ten years time, would we come back to the present to change the way we are today?

Substance and Abuse

Gordon enjoyed a drink. When he was drinking he thought that other people enjoyed him. He also enjoyed the occasional snort of cocaine.

He knew that he was the life and soul of every party, although invitations were getting less frequent than they had been.

He believed that women loved him for his suave wit and perfect dress sense, although they were often elusive in order to stop other women from being too jealous of their relationship with him. He wondered if they might be worried that his dalliances might upset his wife, but there was no need to worry because she had left him a few months before. He had only smacked her gently after she told him that he was drunk. He was not, he was fully in control. He had, it is true, driven his car into another one earlier that same day but the two occurrences were just coincidences.

Anyway, when he had told her that she was fat and unattractive he only wanted to protect her from predatory men who might want to take advantage of her poor mental state. And, a black eye was hardly the most endearing makeup for a woman to wear. The man she had left him for must have been blind or desperate.

Gordon knew that when he drank he seemed to enter

another room. He enjoyed it there. The colours were bright, the gloom of everyday life disappeared. His friends who enjoyed a similar lifestyle were always there to share a story with, although some seemed hard of hearing as they often asked him to repeat what he had said.

Some friends were a little aggressive. They could not hold their drink as well as he could. He knew that because he would sometimes wake up with bruises and scratches and a headache where, probably, somebody had, in fun, hit him.

Gordon enjoyed the special room so much that he planned his life to spend as much time in it as possible. He had lost his job after he had, in fun, grabbed the breasts of one of the girls in the office. He knew she liked him but seemed to have lost her sense of humour on that day and complained to HR.

He thought that she was ugly anyway and should have been grateful for his attention. He told his friends who all agreed that he had been the victim of a huge injustice. "Have another glass of cheer and forget it", they encouraged. He did exactly that, his memory was not as good as it had been in any case.

He had lots of good buddies in the room. One of them knew the secret of life and often sat, beer can in hand, on the streets telling passers by what they needed to know. Sadly, he was unaware that they never understood what he was saying. "Bloody foreigners don't even speak English" he told Gordon although

Gordon could not understand what had been said.

One of Gordon's girlfriends lived in the bright and light room. Even though she had no teeth and seemed to fall over quite a lot, she was good company. She never noticed that he was unable to make love, or have sex as he called it, because she almost always fell asleep as Gordon groped around her body.

He loved her so much that he was quite happy to increase her pleasure in life by sharing her with his friends.

Sometimes, out of nostalgia, he would give her a smack or a punch and she never reacted in the same way that his wife had. She was perfect for him.

The car that knocked Gordon over was the best thing in his life. Two broken legs and two broken arms were, at first, an inconvenience. He was unable to find the entrance to his room. He had to stay in the gloom of normal existence. However, the longer he stayed there the brighter it got.

None of his friends visited him in hospital apart from one. The philosopher had been admitted with chronic liver failure but was still able to tell the doctors and nurses how their lives had gone wrong. They never understood him, and would never until the day they died. The man, beating them to it, died the following day, still misunderstood.

Gordon, now sober, saw the world as it is. The special

room was beginning to look darker as a destination and real life more attractive. He decided to stay where he was and never go into the room again.

It took strength, it took fortitude but he got to where he needed to be and that was where he still is.

Life is more blissful and fulfilling in its reality rather than in an artificial world that is full of vipers that dance seductively before they get close enough to strike that final bite.

The Drunken Truth

In our world of jealous cries,
In our world of tearful eyes,
In this world where sober lies
Are better than the drunken truth.

Now and then we take the chance,
Now and then we kiss and dance,
Until dawn breaks up the trance
That holds us in the drunken truth.

The sober lies that others tell
That honesty is really Hell
And all I do today is sell
My bloodstained heart, the drunken truth.

And now the flush of booze is past
We face the sober truth at last.
Please let the others stand aghast
And teach themselves the drunken truth.

The Sausage and the Ice Cream

Sausages are wonderful if you like them. Sizzling from the grill or straight from the frying pan they are succulent and juicy. Too many can clog your arteries, especially if they contain too much fat. The smell makes us feel hungry and we want to eat them as quickly as we can.

Now, sausages should be a rare treat so when we eat them we should allow their heat to slow us down so that we can enjoy every morsel, every titillation of our taste buds.

Ice cream, on the other hand, is an opposite. It comes from the freezer so it is cold. We need to eat it slowly but quickly enough so it is not melted slush by the time we get to the last mouthful.

This is similar to experiences. We should enjoy every moment of every event in our lives. We have to match the pace at which we consume our day-by-day happenings whether they are hot or cold. Too many, or too much, can be bad for us. We need variation. One sensation followed by another.

Yet timing is important. Sausages that are eaten too quickly will burn us. Ice cream eaten too quickly will freeze our tongues.

Life and its experiences, the encounters with fate, should be taken at the correct pace. We can be hungry for change, we can be too greedy for the same old things but we should enjoy the differences. Quiet solitude is enjoyable when followed by hustle and bustle.

Frantic behaviour is wonderful when we have time to reflect upon what we have done.

Sweet and savoury; hot and cold; spicy or bland. These are all in the compass of our senses of taste.

We should strive to obtain the same counterpoints in our lives for maximum enjoyment.

Whatever life brings we need to savour every moment, bitter or sweet.

Growing Up, Growing Down

Brigetta was a small girl. She was the youngest of three children who lived in the house. She had one older brother and one older sister.

Her siblings seemed favoured until Brigetta was born. Her brother, the first born was seen as the child from Heaven, the son, the heir, the apple of his mother's eye.

When the next child was born everybody was delighted it was a girl. No competition for the brother, no competition for the mother and she became the Princess the father wanted in his family.

So life was blissful until Brigetta was born.

The existing Princess felt that she had been sent into exile. The father had a new Princess, the mother a new baby to dote on and the brother was bored by the two girls.

He would pick on Brigetta as she grew. His first sister was too close to him in size and would fight back if challenged.

The sister would take out her annoyance with her younger sibling as she was stronger.

Brigetta dreamed of becoming bigger so that she would make more of a presence in the home. She needed to be bigger in order to survive so she ate.

Her parents loved their chubby daughter and spoilt her by buying sweets and chocolate. Brigetta got bigger. Not in height but in girth. The fat she carried helped to protect her from the occasional punch from her brother and the more frequent punches from her sister.

When she started school, Brigetta was as heavy as her older sister but shorter. Her new class mates saw that she was plump and ignored it. However, one day, a year after they had first met and after the summer break, Brigetta was becoming huge. One girl called her Brigetta Bigeater and the name stuck.

Boys would bully her and called her names. She never had a boyfriend, unlike her sister who was able to add name after name to her list of admirers.

Brigetta, in her early teens, did meet boys who wanted to find a girl who was easy to please. They would use her and leave her. As parting comments they would often tell her how gross she was and that nobody would ever want to be with her. She was so very big by now.

Her dream had come to be, but at a high price. No boys or men would want to be near her so she was safe. Her true love was chocolate but sadly, her enemy was the same thing.

When Brigetta was at her school she had a classmate. They did not really know each other but their lives were connected by food.

Ann was a young and happy girl when she started school but there was a sad day awaiting her.

She was innocent until the age of eight. Sometimes a neighbour was asked to look after her while her parents went out and they became good friends. He would buy her presents and she enjoyed it when her parents went out. She stayed up late watching the television with William.

This was a perfect childhood until one night something happened. William turned out to be a child molester. He did nasty things and threatened Ann that all sorts of bad things would happen if she told.

Ann wanted to remain innocent but that was no longer possible. She buried the memory until, when she was in her early teenage years; a boy was too forceful with her. This was rape rather than seduction. Ann was mortified. She decided somewhere in her head that the safest place to be was in her earlier childhood. She refused to get bigger. She stopped eating and stayed at the same weight for a few years. Even this did not stop the looks she received from men and so she started losing weight. She was going to be the same size as she was at eight, the real safe place for her to be before the troubles started.

One of her classmates, the same person who gave the

nickname to Brigetta, started to call her Ann O'Wrecks-it. Such is the creative cruelty of some children.

It was years later when Brigetta and Ann met at an eating disorder clinic. One was to lose weight, the other to gain it.

Being bigger comes from being taller rather than fatter. The way to overcome bullying is from being stronger and fitter rather than being the object of ridicule that maintains the problem.

On the other hand, being smaller never preserves the innocence of a child in the adult. Rather than punishing the body that Ann held responsible for the abuse she needed to punish the perpetrators of the abuse. Let <u>them</u> suffer rather than the victim.

PS. Ann and Brigetta are pretty much the same size as each other now and became the best of friends.

The Bullied Bully

Margaret was a bully. She bullied other girls at school including Brigetta and Ann. She loved her job. She would go to school and her creativity was spent on devising names for her peers that reflected her view of how they were.

Anyone with acne, ginger hair, glasses or a speech impediment would be at the mercy of Margaret's taunts.

She felt good, she had control of her life. When she returned home her mother insisted that she cleaned and cooked. There was too much on daytime TV that would be missed otherwise. Her mother loved the programmes that highlighted the sad lives of others. She would shout and scream her opinion at the hosts of the 'shows'. In them she could see her own life being described. Her husband was a drunken womaniser who never gave any emotion other than anger to his family.

When he arrived home he would argue, he would hit and he would assert his role as the alpha male in this pack of humans. Margaret was always close to his fist when he used it, although he would never let the results be in public view. A deft punch to the kidneys, a poke in the stomach would suffice. Margaret wanted to retaliate but she was too young and her father too big. Her mother would never step him because she carried enough of his bruises to be fearful of trying to help.

Margaret had no outlet for her fears and her hurts apart from the other girls at school.

The words she used reflected those that were used at home. If somebody has spots it was because they were dirty and should be cleaned up. If they were overweight it was because they were too lazy to do exercise.

Spectacle wearers wasted too much time with their heads stuck in books and so on and on.

Margaret needed a strong man in her life to protect her from the wrath of her father. She had lots of boyfriends as if she were on a quest to find a suitable partner.

She left school as soon as he was able and used the little money she saved from her wages, after her father had taken a huge share, to buy clothes, makeup and perfumes to attract the man of her dreams.

She found one. His name was Tony. He liked life and he was a fun man to be with. In some respects he reminded her of her father. She thought she would fight fire with fire. She needed a man who could look after himself and her. However, Tony became too much like her father and his angry outbursts. He bullied her to extremes. He called her names, abused her body and made her life a total misery, again.

The irony is plain to see.

Losing Your Temper

Margaret's husband Tony, certainly looked after himself but care for others was not in his remit at that moment, but became so when Margaret threatened to leave him. That had never been an option in her younger years at her parent's house.

Tony looked for help. He came to realise that his anger was not so much about frightening other people, but it had been a protection against his own vulnerability.

He had no reason to scare the people he loved so much, but he desperately wanted to prevent being hurt. It was as if he wanted to bully the people that he loved into loving him. He knew that this was foolish. It is the sort of thing that children do. They threaten to run away, or to hurt themselves in the hope that they will be found or made a fuss of.

It made him think of the times he had threatened to hurt or kill himself. He had often told Margaret that he would allow himself to be killed by some of the violent people he mixed with. He knew that threats like that never worked. Bullies only build hatred rather than love.

He had never thought of himself as a bully before. It was not necessary to hit people in order to be a bully. Words were as potent a weapon as a fist or a cudgel. The purpose was the same. To change somebody else's point of view by force rather than persuasion or negotiation.

It was always a selfish act, using strength of force or volume of language to win. Negotiation is about both sides getting what they need and want, within reason. Bullying is not about reason, it is an irrational act of violence. The reasonable man will listen to the other's words and respond with open-minded intelligence.

Negotiation is like love in that it is almost an act of mutual seduction. Love was the thing that seemed to be denied to Tony. Perhaps that is why he could now perceive of himself as having been a verbal and physical bully.

He wanted love and his only way forward was to give it rather than to demand it by threat.

With the help he was given, Tony started to wonder what anger was. He had heard about the so-called fight-or-flight response so he thought that if an angry person runs away then that is survival rather than cowardice. This included the survival of the emotion of love as well as the physical form.

His conclusion was that anger was also about fighting or self-protection. Yet, the real outcome was that of loss; not of the fight but the quality of his life. The question was how could he control it?

Given the choice between running away from conflict or fighting the perceived cause of it, then the answer was difficult for him. But with thought and consideration of the consequences, the choice became an easier one to make.

In the past, when his Margaret said something that he disagreed with then he certainly would not run away. She would take that as his sign of weakness. He would only have the option of fighting her. Mostly with words but sometimes with his hands.

If using words, he could shout as if scaring a rabbit from his lettuces. That was a form of fighting but the rabbit never fought back. Sometimes he would shout as if scaring something more hostile like a fierce and growling dog.

If using his hands it could be like waving a mosquito away or something more aggressive such as a wasp that would be squashed.

None of those things were his wife, however. She was a gentle soul who offered little threat.

Now, not a lot of words are devoted to the passive elements of the fight-or-flight response, namely defend or freeze.

The answer he had sought was contained within these other responses. If he became angry then he could utilize defending his point without anger. So if his wife told him he should cut the grass he would explain why he had not rather than getting angry with her perceived nagging. Then he could tell her that he would do it the following day. She would then smile and give him a hug.

He had the other choice of freezing, controlling himself so that he could look to a calm conversation and yet another hug. This took time to learn and his wife took time to learn that he had learnt and for her to regain trust. She had been at the point where her only option had been to run from the angry man. Now she could help him to repair and heal.

The bad temper that Tony had was now being lost, but in a totally different way.

Angry people have the choice between remaining angry and losing everything or learning that control, patience and peace are a far better option for happiness in their lives. This is never giving in to a person but gaining the upper hand over their own angry behaviour.

Look at the double meaning in the phrase "losing your temper". This can be seen as becoming angry...or losing the cause of the loss of control.

Change

In order to escape the familiar scenes that surrounded me, I drove my car to the coast. I booked into a cheap hotel with a view inland rather than over the sea, which was what I had wanted. It was the penalty for taking one of the few rooms remaining. I looked at the greenery of the landscape which seemed to take my focus to a small stunted tree at the top of a hill. I could sympathise with it. It was sad, alone and exposed.

Later, I went shopping for clothes. I knew that buying a new wardrobe was an attempt to change the outer 'me' so that my inner self would, hopefully, follow suit.

The afternoon was spent walking along the beach. It was early in the Spring so there few people to share it with. I thought that I would treat myself to an expensive meal in the evening. Economies of scale are wonderful when you are alone. For the price of two meals, I could indulge myself completely. I booked a table for eight o'clock at a beach-side restaurant and returned to my hotel. There was a comedy show on the television and I found myself laughing loudly for the first time in months.

I bathed, dressed and admired myself in the full-length mirror in my room. It was like being sixteen again, not knowing what the night would hold for me. It was a feeling of re-birth. A new me would walk into the world with his head held high. I had worn my old clothes for far too long.

The food was good. Sea-bass washed down with Chablis. On top of that, I deposited a chocolate pudding with cream. Two brandies were added and it was all left to marinade in my stomach.

I walked to the beach after my meal. The stars were bright in the dark sky. Their light seemed to be reflected by the mass of tiny shells that sat on the damp sand at the water's edge. Perhaps it was the wine, but I could imagine the beach to be the sky and the sky to be beneath my feet. There was a sense of silence in the night which was an oasis in the continuing noises of modern life.

The constant roar of automobiles, the ever present jet engines overhead. Those interruptions had ceased to be at that point of time.

The movement of the sea as it reached to caress the beach sounded like the planet breathing its sighs of resignation to its apparent domination by mankind. I stood, watched and listened for as long as was needed to make me feel that I was of no more importance to the Universe than one of the shells on that beach. Surprisingly, I found the thought to be reassuring.

I walked back to the hotel, undressed and hung up my new clothes. I felt mellow. Even the reflux that I felt when I went to bed seemed worthwhile. My sleep was, once again, dream free.

I woke at ten o'clock. However, the reflection of the smart man I had seen the evening before had turned into that of my father. The thought of breakfast was not appealing so I made my way to the beach again. I wandered along the sea edge looking at the stars still resting in the sand. I looked at, and sometimes picked up small white pebbles. Without any reason, I crammed the stones that had attracted my attention into my pockets.

There were cliffs which watched the sea with a stern sense of duty. The ocean could be an unruly child at times when it was being encouraged by the wind, but most of the time it was gentle and well behaved.

The cliffs had layers of different colours which fascinated me. Structures were representing time through different stages.

They were as the layers that seemed to be observable in my life. They were the strata that told the story of my life through its troubled history to this moment of tranquillity at the coast, and to my existence on my own in my new haven.

And life shows through the separate stories. Each layer is different, yet they all constituted me, as the different levels made up the essence of the cliff.

I packed my old clothes into the bag that my new ones had been in, settled my account ; dropped my old life off at a Charity Shop, and drove back to my new reality.

The Saloon Car and The Sports Model.

Esse quam videre.
(To be, is better than to seem to be.)

Joseph had a family, a house and a car.

The car was a steady, safe and reliable saloon that offered security for his family, but he thought it was boring.

"Won't be long before I'm driving along with a hat and a pipe while wearing my slippers." He would say in a sarcastic way to his wife.

He had a good job but not good enough for him to afford two cars. He wanted, he dreamed, of a faster model that would impress rather than be looked down on.

Secretly he saved. He held onto money that he should have used for house repairs, school uniforms and general maintenance of his home and family.

And one day he decided that he had saved enough to buy a sports car.

It had two small seats and one large engine. It was red and made a purring sound when sitting at traffic lights and the roar of a lion as he pulled away.

Sandra's car had broken down by the side of the road.

Joseph, while driving around on a Saturday afternoon saw this lady in distress and pulled over.

"Do you need some help?" he asked.

"Yes please. The car has stopped and I cannot get it started again."

Joseph looked at the engine, shook his head and said that it would not be easily repaired. He had actually seen the cause of the problem being quickly mended but he wanted to give this pretty lady a lift.

"Could you drop me off at my home, please? I need to get back to meet my sister."

He agreed even before he knew where she lived. She got into the car as he held the door open for her and admired her long legs.

Asking for directions, he was not disturbed that she lived 50 miles away.

He started the engine. It purred as sweetly as he did. He gunned the engine and set off at speed. They chatted as he drove. She asked him questions and he lied the answers back to her.

He was a big wheel in a company, spend a lot of time overseas, he owned a villa in Florida and was single, of course.

He dropped her off. She said she would call a recovery company to collect her car. They exchanged telephone numbers and he was sure that his description of himself as a successful entrepreneur had hooked her.

She told him that she was a model.

On his return home he explained to his wife that the 'cheap' car he had bought for just a small amount was 'playing up' and that he had broken down.

His wife laughed at his tale not knowing any different.

He met Sandra at increasing regular times. She loved his style and his car.

He worried that his credit card was taking a bigger and bigger strain each month. They were now lovers and he needed to maintain the belief she had that he was a virile man-about-town.

They had to meet in hotels to make love as his penthouse flat was being renovated and her house was being used by her sister as she had got a job that required her to live away from her own home.

Sandra's husband was as suspicious about her days out as was Joseph's wife about his.

They did not know each other but they met in the hotel car park on the day that they had both followed their respective spouses.

They both watched as Sandra and Joseph walked into the hotel lobby hand-in-hand. They both got out of their cars and gesticulated. They looked at each other and after a short pause, laughed.

"Do you mean that you know him?" Sandra's husband asked Joseph's wife.

"Know him? I'm married to the cheating swine. Do you know who the tart is?"

"The tart is my wife" he replied.

After that the two of them started a relationship based on their shared experiences.

When Joseph finally ran out of money and could neither afford insurance and petrol for his car Sandra dumped him. On the same day Sandra's husband dumped her and Joseph's wife dumped him.

The wronged couple were righted as they got together permanently, and happily. They had both found something steady, safe and reliable rather than fast, dangerous and untrustworthy.

Sandra and Joseph never saw each other again. All they found were road-works in their fast lanes

Being what you are is important. Appearing to be what you are not will lead to trouble. As has been said before by wise people; a good liar needs a good memory.

The Court Jester

The jester was fairly bad, to be honest. Among his jokes were lines like, "I have a weak bladder" as he waved his pig's bladder and sprayed the crowd with water.

"Off with his head", the King would cry as the crowd burst into laughter and the jester ran, slowly, to feign fear. The King had the catch phrase rather than the joker.

"Have you heard the one about the chastity belt that the hand-maiden wore? She has a spare key. She hates the days but loves the Knights"

"Off with his head". The crowd roared.

The jester's job was to bring laughter to the Court. His jokes were never funny but the audience loved the banter between him and the King.

"Why did the chicken cross the road?"

"Axe me another" the King would shout.

The courtiers joined in. "Off with his head."

The astrologer was jealous. He never got laughs; he never had a response from the King that was amusing. He was jealous of the jester's relationship with the

King.

He had a plan, however. At the next meeting of the Oval Table he would make a forecast that would take away the laughter and set gloom over the Kingdom. That would mean he would get more attention and his wise advice would be sought.

"At the last full-moon the stars showed me that famine and disease will come to the Kingdom. Many will suffer, many will die. What I saw decreed that all laughter should be banned. The sound of jollity annoys the planets and they are sending punishment to mankind. We have to ensure that not one joke is told, not one person falls into the moat and not one Knight falls off his horse."

The advisors and supporters of the throne were silent. Some held their giggles at the idea of Knights coming off horses. The jester had used the line that "Knight is falling" about Sir Cumference, a rather portly man and a bad horseman.

"When does this all start?" asked the King.

"It will happen when the sun is made dark by the moon next week. I will make the moon move away from the sun after I have received a thousand gold coins to appease the planets and they will give us relief from the punishment."

The fortune teller was bad at most things but he had been told about solar eclipses by Ma Lynne, a witch who made a living by selling charms and curses.

She had started a relationship with the astrologer after he had ensured that she would never be burnt at the stake by predicting that if she were then the sky would be covered in ash for ever.

At the appointed hour the following week the sun started to disappear behind the moon. It got darker and darker until the sun vanished.

"Magician, do your magic, bring the sun back." The King had a tone of panic in his voice. You will receive your gold coins.

At that moment, the astrologer stepped back, partly from shock and partly for dramatic effect. He and his wand fell backwards into the moat. He was silenced by the blow to his head from a log that had been floating there.

It took longer to resuscitate him than it did for the eclipse to end. The confidence trick was exposed at the same time as the sun.

"He didn't get a chance to cast his spell. He is a fraud." Said the King.

Everybody was happy that the plague and famine would not happen.

The jester stepped forward and said, "Did you see the astrologer fall in the moat. He didn't see that one coming." The crowd laughed.

"Off with his head," said the King.

Nobody was laughing.

The King was pointing at the astrologer. The look on his face said that he meant it this time.

Mythology and Fortune Telling

Fortune telling rests on the idea that the future is predictable as if written in a film script or by a divine entity who has nothing better to do. It is not.

However people make money from giving the impression that the future can be predicted by their ability to read signs and omens.

Astrology relies heavily on the input from the many different positions of planets and stars that allow a truly infinite number of possible interpretations. Each planet is given its own character and its own sphere of influence. That these influences are real is unlikely. It has never been proved that there are any major measurable effects from the planets that could alter human behaviour. What did astrologers do when Pluto turned out to be a nebulous bunch of rock and gas?

The key has to rest with subjective interpretation.

One human is making statements about another or himself using astrology as a technique for giving stimulation for thought.

For example, if you are in a happy relationship and you read in your horoscope, "Today, you will meet the person of your dreams", then if you are meeting your partner for dinner, you would be happy. However, if you meet a really nice person during the course of the day then you might be predisposed to view that person in a different way that might just damage your existing relationship. The words in the horoscope remain the same, but the outcome could be changed by your own introspective interpretation of those words.

How about if you read your partner's horoscope and it says that they will meet a secret admirer and find love? Does that lead to love or turmoil in your relationship?

This seems to be the explanation of books such as 'I-Ching'. Vague answers are given that need to be interpreted in the context of the question asked. The information comes from the mind of the enquirer, however. This is not to denigrate the wisdom of the I-Ching, but rather to admire the psychological techniques that the writer employed way back in time. Before a question is asked of the oracle, the questioner has to work out the wording. Intent is added that gives direction to the message obtained.

For another example, take the process of reading tea-leaves. The tea-leaves do not foretell the future but the reader perhaps appears to. It requires taking input and the creative 'interpretation' of that 'information' from a personal point of view.

The drawback of fortune telling is that they attach values to inanimate objects that are within the positive-to-negative range. For example, the Ace of Spades has many negative associations.

Most fortune telling techniques using playing cards use at least seven cards. In a pack of fifty two cards, therefore, there is just about a seven to one chance of reading a hand including the ace of spades, (that is 7 cards from 52). If consulted daily then the card will appear, by chance, once per week. Bearing in mind that people tend to want their fortunes told when things are going badly rather than well, because they are looking for relief, that frequency of occurrence of a negative sign will probably do more harm than good.

It is easier to my mind to approach a problem with a good creative plan, rather than waiting for a planet to move!

Battles have been lost because generals have fought them with the negative omens from the entrails of goats affecting their ability to think rationally. Better luck must have ridden with the generals who planned all possibilities with a free, open and creative mind.

If you want to see the future then make it happen. Plan the future, let your plans unfold. Superstition prevents you from doing things. Hope and optimism will create confidence in YOUR ability to make an outcome happen, never the stars, tealeaves, coffee grounds, ladders, cracks in the paving slabs...do I need to go on?

No.

The Genie in the Bottle

Way back in time, in a strange land, a genie was put into a bottle because he created malevolence and caused pain to humans. He became very angry and swore to get revenge on humankind.

He was very subtle and liked to hide before jumping out when the bottle was opened, and causing chaos and havoc.

He was seductive in the way he worked. He smiled through the glass and made women want him. He smiled charmingly at men and made them want him. He was a genie who could change at will.

When he was given freedom then he would promise success and hilarity to the wish maker. He would bring memories back and allow the person to reminisce about times in their pasts.

These seemed like good wishes to give but the genie was cursed to see freedom for a while but then he would be trapped again. The magician who had him placed in his prison was very adept at creating spells.

Part of this bitterness at being trapped was built into the behaviour of the genie. He would crave liberation and make all sorts of promises to men and women but his real aim was to replace himself in the bottle with the soul of humans.

After smiling, after bringing laughter, after nearly being out of his trap...he would pounce.

He would make the human do things that no human should do. He would make the person shout, punch and scream. He would make the person feel so confident that they would drive cars recklessly whilst thinking they were as good as anybody.

They would be made to kill; they would be made to try to rape.

They became as bad as the genie. Their souls, their self-esteem would be open for the grabs made by the little and corrupted essence of badness.

However, the magician saw what had been created and decided to place another genie in the bottle. This one was able to fight the evil one but never destroy it. It gave the ability to stop. It gave control.

In every bottle of alcohol that is available, those two genies live. There is a dividing line hidden in the liquid. At the top the good genie is there to give a sense of relaxation but below that line the bad genie takes over.

All people who drink alcohol can make the wish that the good genie will tell them when to stop drinking to avoid getting to the level where it cannot control the evil one.

The good genie can make that wish come true. However those people who relish releasing the evil genie will find that after the enjoyment of the company of the good one then they have to face the evil and nasty one who takes over without warning. As said before, it is a subtle creature.

That genie makes people suffer. It enjoys destroying relationships, careers, family life and it gets a huge buzz from killing people through drunken driving, fighting or illness.

If you drink alcohol, be aware of the two genies and never take the chance of meeting the bad one. This is about knowing limits when drinking. If you have let the bad genie out, then perhaps you need to get help from somebody who can put the cork back in the bottle and throw it away. When you see the behaviour of people in holiday resorts or weekend bars who drink to the point where they lose control, lose self respect and allow things to happen that would shock the members of a Roman orgy; then you can see that magicians curse in full flow.

The Puff-Adder

The woman screamed. Her son was looking in bewildered enthralment at the puff-adder as it slithered along.

As if evaluating the risk it stared at the young boy. Its tongue flickered in and out. It hissed and made a half-hearted strike, more to frighten than to kill. The boy ran away, followed by his mother who needed to still his sobs and dry his tears.

At the age of two he did not know the difference between a real threat and a fascinating creature that had no legs.

The Namibian desert is a hostile place that is home to the Kalahari bush-men. These men and women live in a place that has little food and less drink. Over the thousands of years that they have lived there they have developed a relationship with the land. They will only kill to eat after they have asked permission from the spirits.

So this young lad had a lot to learn about the animals and meagre resources that gave his kin life.

The puff-adder lived in their territory. It had a right to be there, but it had to hunt to feed itself on the scarce supplies. The venom in its fangs had to be potent as there were no second chances. This valuable poison was held in reserve and it was a last resort in defence, hence the young boy's life being saved. As a first strike weapon, however, it was perfect. The rats it lived on were fast and had to be stopped in their tracks.

When the young lad was in his early teenage years, he was taken hunting by his father and other men. He had hunted with them before but on this occasion he saw his second puff-adder. The snake saw the men and watched as they approached. It prepared its defence against the threat.

The now young man saw it and started to panic. The men with him laughed. They explained that the puff-adder, when handled with respect, made a good dinner. They approached it, distracted it, and with one fatal throw of a spear, beheaded it. Prayers were offered to the spirit of the snake and it was wished well in its new life

After the body had stopped writhing it was picked up, slung over a shoulder and carried until it was time to eat.

It was good. The men told stories as they sat around their fire. They explained that things can be a threat to a child and the fear it causes will live in the child for ever. Yet, if care is taken then the source of that fear can be transmuted into a vital resource. The hunger of these men had been satisfied by the snake.

Respect and caution were vital in catching it but fear would have been dangerous because hesitation or sudden moves would have provoked retaliation.

Fears are necessary for protection but these wise men knew that fear should have limits. Unless change is made then suffering will follow. Change can be made when the child becomes old enough to be able to see through its natural safety blanket.

This story refers to things like spiders that are normally harmless but which can create fear. This comes from our early days and probably go back to our human hardwiring from our primeval heritage when they were more threatening. Those fears are known as atavistic phobias and can apply to those things that were potentially dangerous in our history such as snakes, lizards, frogs, spiders to name but a few.

Our modern world is far safer and we should follow the example in the story. Many of those things we fear help us by eating the real threats. Lizards, frogs and spiders eat flies and mosquitoes. Snakes eat rats and mice. Within our fears we should look for the goodness in those things we seem to hate.

The Twelve Year Old Pilot

Trevor got onto the passenger aircraft and made himself comfortable. He was flying to a remote island for a holiday with his wife and two children.

Having placed his bag in the overhead locker, He watched the other passengers do the same.

The captain came on the speaker system. "Good morning ladies and gentlemen. We have a slight delay before take-off so we will leave the doors open for added ventilation. I hope that we will soon be given clearance for take-off. I hope you enjoy your flight with Metaphor Airlines. While we are waiting for clearance, let me tell you a few things about the flight. My name is Ben and I am your pilot. I am twelve years old and I have been flying for a couple of hours. Even though I have little, or no, experience I am happy to take you to your destination."

The man grabbed his wife and children and headed to the door fighting through the growing crowd of passengers who wanted to get off.

In that moment of panic, Trevor's life flashed before him. He remembered the time that he had been forced to stand at the front of his school class and deliver a talk about the breeding cycle of chimpanzees. He was embarrassed at the thought beforehand. The idea of giving information about sexual encounters between creatures very much like humans was too similar to what he had been told about the facts of life by his mother. This made him want to run away. In front of the class he sweated, he panted, he felt dizzy. He would have been alright talking about frogs or bees, but...

The experience made him react in the same way if ever he was asked to make a speech, give a presentation or in any way appear in a public theatre.

After a while Trevor's mind returned to the situation on the aircraft. All passengers were told that there was now a different pilot, an older man. Boarding the plane for the second time the sense of relief was immense for all passengers.

The pilot came on the speaker system. "Good morning ladies and gentlemen. We have a slight delay before take-off so we will leave the doors open for added ventilation. I hope that we will soon be given clearance for take-off. I hope you enjoy your flight with Metaphor Airlines. While we are waiting for clearance, let me tell you a few things about the flight. My name is Gregory and I am your pilot. I am thirty five years old and I have been flying for many years."

This man, the same age as Trevor, was somebody all the passengers could trust.

Gregory continued. "The reason that you would not let a twelve year old fly you to a blissful destination is that you would not believe that he had enough life experience to make decisions about what to do. As this is Metaphor Airlines, let me give you the meaning of this story.

We have a man on board called Trevor. When he was twelve years old he was in a situation that need careful handling, an emergency. He had to cope and found that he did not have enough experience to do so. He did what you feared that Ben, our twelve year old pilot, would do. He crashed. Now at the tender age of thirty five Trevor's mind is still being flown by the twelve year old pilot in his head. He has twenty three years of experience of decision making and knowledge in his head. The things that you all hope that I have. Through this story I want Trevor to stop being controlled by a twelve year old. Accept that life has moved on and that you are able to cope."

With that, Trevor got out of his seat, made his way to the front of the plane and delivered a heart-touching speech about the mating cycle of chimpanzees. His breathing was calm, his speech paced to allow people to understand what was being said and his delivery was animated. He did miss out some parts of the animation, however!

He walked back to his seat to the sound of rapturous applause.

There is a young pilot in all of us who needs to be allowed to grow into a person who can cope in the situations we find ourselves in our later years.

Elementary Truth

Like a huge whale after a harpoon strike, our planet reeled and shook at the pain caused by the people. Its cries were heard far and wide but the men wanted all that could be taken.

In the same way that the whale would be cut to pieces to provide fat for fuel, meat for food, skin for leather and its bones for whatever, the planet was being dissected for its resources.

The planet, not being stupid but lacking a voice that could persuade humans, decided to react. It had a meeting with the four elements.

Air wanted to be cleaner. It wanted pollution to subside. It needed to nurture the plants and animals. It gave the breath of life but, with the exhaust fumes and factory plumes, that breath had a smell of rank halitosis.

Earth wanted to stop the continual bleeding as men sucked out its oil. They carved out its metal and precious stones. Why were these so precious anyway? Gem stones were mostly for adornment. They had no real value other than enhancing the appearance of the people who wore them. Men died mining these things for little return. The profit was for the dealers and traders. Land was laid bare to make profits paid in paper made from the trees in the rain forests. Precious things? Ivory was precious because it came from big creatures such as elephants, although nobody seemed to realise that the elephant is the most precious thing rather than its tusk. Rhinoceros horn was regarded as an aphrodisiac because it really belonged to a creature perceived as dangerous and that was decorated by a phallic symbol! People are strange!

Water needed to be respected and to be cleaned up. The seas were used as dumps for the leftovers from the Earth. Nuclear fuels, plastics, sewage, mercury and all sorts of things that harmed. They were thought to be safer in the sea because they became invisible to humans. They polluted the lives of the fish and other life forms in the sea. It destroyed the plankton that fed the fish and gave oxygen back to the air. These little plants trapped carbon dioxide as they floated on the surface. Plankton gave nourishment to the whales that were being hunted.

Fire was blamed for pollution. Without fire there would be no jet engines, car engines, furnaces or factories. Precious metals could not be melted. Fire was the culprit it was decided. It took oxygen from the air and returned carbon dioxide.

The four elements held their meeting and unlike so many human committee meetings, it came to a course of action.

The Planet vomited as a volcano. **Fire** made the lava be as hot as possible. **Earth** added sand and silica to make a dust. **Water** added ice crystals to make the cloud all but invisible and finally **Air** blew the cloud towards the inhabited areas of the planet.

They chose the parts of the planet that were causing trouble. The parts where air transport was a way of life; where the people would be made immovable by chaos.

Elsewhere on the planet, at the same time, there were earthquakes, monsoons, hurricanes and fires. The planet was screaming at a loud and high pitch. Would the people listen? Would they stop flying food from parts of the world where it was grown by hungry people but flown to other countries for profit?

Would people think about different communication methods other than personal meetings after flying thousands of miles?

Would fish stocks be preserved by slowing the mass destruction of fish?

Mankind had to learn that the elements can be asked to help life but when they are used as slaves then they will fight back with strength and with a fierceness that cannot be tamed.

The Elements of Monkton Wyld

*We circled close in morning **Air**,*
Sweet singing in the round.
Unity for self and all.
Sublime, inspiring sound.

*On **Earth**'s soft, damp and gentle face,*
We sat and sang our part,
I looked into your eyes of peace
That showed your depth of heart.

*And **Water** shed from those deep eyes,*
Sad tears of hurt and wrong
Were turned to joy and happiness,
That shone brightly in your song.

***Fire** that glowed from deep within*
Gave heat to your warm smile.
Giving so much loving beauty,
That endures beyond that while.

*****

Author's Note: Monkton Wyld Court is a centre for sustainable living near Dorset's Jurassic Coast. As well as workshops and family weeks, they teach skills for sustainable living: beekeeping, permaculture, eco-building, green technologies, sustainable land use and environmental crafts.

http://www.monktonwyldcourt.co.uk/

The Vanity of Power

Jordan was getting ready for the conference.

His wife ironed his shirts, pressed his pants and socks as she watched the TV.

Jordan cleaned his teeth with his electric toothbrush. He enjoyed the routine of the morning. Ten minutes in the power shower followed by careful preening with the powerful bathroom lights shining on his face. He looked for spots; he searched for areas of his face that his electric razor might have missed.

After dressing and eating his breakfast, he packed his bag, kissed his wife and son and then got into his car. Jordan was an important man in his business so he had the big, luxurious car that showed his status to anybody and everybody who saw him in it.

The car growled its way into life and Jordan was on his way.

"Where is Dad going, mum?"

"Well, darling; he is going to the airport and then he is flying in the company jet to meet some people for a conference. He is going to be nearly half way around the World."

"Will he be gone long?"

"Just a week or so. Anyway I have heated your milk for your cereals for your breakfast. Eat up and I will drive you to school. I need to drop you off and come back to get myself ready for my run on the treadmill that Daddy bought me. It saves me running in the park and it has so many bits to it that I don't know how to work yet."

The mother and son got into her 4X4 car and started the half mile drive to the school.

"Why does dad have to be away for so long?"

"Well, son. The conference is for one day, the travelling will take two days and daddy wants to do some driving around and he wants to hire a speed boat so he can relax a bit. He works very hard."

"What is the conference about, mum?"

"It is about energy conservation. We all need to cut back on wasting energy so that we can have a better future. When the oil runs out then we will have to find different energy sources if we want to live good lives. Daddy and I do our best to save energy, don't we? We do our bit. That is why daddy has gone all that way for his conference. Anyway, I will pick you up later, OK?"

"But mum, I am 11 years old. My friends think I am lazy."

"Don't be silly. What is the point in having a car if you do not use it? Besides, you need to save your strength so you can learn all about how we can do our best to conserve energy."

The boy climbed out of the car and waddled into his school. He had saved enough energy as a fat store to keep him warm and snug. He had enough to ensure he would never starve if the production of food ceased.

His mother was very proud of her family and the efforts they were making to ensure the survival of the planet.

Sometimes we do things that are ludicrous. Ironing shirts throughout the Western world takes the resources of electricity and time for an expression that is nothing more than vanity. Running on a treadmill that is powered is a strange alternative to running in the open air. Driving big cars and driving short distances also panders to vanity and laziness. Flying to a conference about energy conservation is a poor alternative to video conferences. Not only fuel is saved, so is time, a precious thing as well. Power, or energy, is a finite resource. Wasting it needlessly is so destructive.

Profit and Loss

Richard slid into the smooth and soft leather seat, fastened his seat-belt, sat back as the engine started and began his journey.

As he drove away to the airport, he waved to Helen, his wife.

After he had boarded the executive jet he slid into the smooth and soft leather seat, fastened his seat belt, sat back as the engines started and began his journey.

As the plane taxied to the runway he asked his pretty PA if she had everything that he needed for his meeting.

He was about to travel to a conference in Aruba. He enjoyed the time he spent making money as a high-earning, high-flying executive of a highly profitable bank.

He made so much money in bonuses that his biggest problem, he thought, was how to spend it all.

The luxury house he lived in, from time to time, was paid for. His son and daughter had the best possible education that money could buy. They boarded at the best schools and every-so-often they would write letters home to tell their parents what had been happening.

Yes, Richard was a very successful man. His advice was worth a fortune.

He would tell potential investors that they could make the choice between profit and loss. They could borrow money from his bank that would aid their cash flow. Money borrowed would buy equipment that was needed for their growth. They could take over other companies to expand their bases, and so on.

The business of business kept Richard busy. He was so absorbed by his work that he had to make time by cancelling his promises to attend functions at his children's schools. He never saw his son playing sports for the first teams he belonged to. He never saw his daughter perform the lead roles in the plays she was the star of.

When they left school and went to University, he was unable to take them to where they would be living. He was able to pay for their educations, however, and that made him happy.

Richard was away on business for both their graduations. He missed the ceremonies but he saw the photographs of his loved ones in their gowns and mortar boards.

His children got good jobs and started to earn substantial salaries at around the time that Richard had his first heart attack. Both his children were too busy to visit him in hospital but they did ask their PA's to sent cards wishing him a swift recovery. Richard's wife did visit him from time to time but found that she was trying to talk to a stranger. The conversation was all small-talk and she was relieved when she joined her paramour afterwards. He was a man who, in money terms was poor. He was a man, however, who could show an interest in Helen. He gave her compliments and love. He cherished this woman who, up until he had met her, had been like a lone rose in the desert; a beauty in an unseeing prison.

Richard demanded computer support in his bed but this was disallowed by the consultant who was looking after him. Even threats to have him dismissed, after all Richard had paid a huge amount in private health insurance, failed to get him what he wanted.

He had no option but to lay in his bed pondering his life. He had suspicions about the possibility that Helen was having an affair so his Private Investigator had investigated and broke the news to him. Divorce was the next step to take but that would reduce his value by half and that was unthinkable. Better to take the cheaper option of letting his wife be occupied with her own interests while Richard could work, and whenever he needed he could and would buy the comforts of young ladies in whichever town he was staying in. His PA had now left his employ and had settled down in a new job that was less demanding in all respects.

Life had been difficult for Richard. He had been required to make choices. He had to choose his career path. He had to choose a wife who would be happy with the lonely times when he was away. He had to make decisions that would affect the lives of the winners and losers he dealt with. It made little difference to him because in order to make profits he knew somebody had to make a loss to keep the whole thing in balance. His life was like a gigantic creature that had to consume others. He crushed what got in his way and gave short term benefits to those who could assist his own journey.

Yet now he was alone. The pretty girls he had bought were off the market in his sterile bed in the intensive care unit. The bottles of champagne and wine that cost as much as a small country needed for health care were off-limits.

Why should he care? Soon he would be back on the road again making his deals.

Very few people attended his funeral. The business colleagues that he had known were too busy making their deals. His wife and children were there but his son had to attend a meeting the next day so he left early. His daughter was due to fly to Australia to clinch a deal. His wife had to show her devotion as a widow so she had to take a cruise to overcome the shock. Much to the amazement of her friends, on that sailing she met a nice man who would keep her company. They met whilst dining in the first-class lounge.

Certainly it was a pretence, but Helen had to keep up the appearance of a dutiful wife so her meeting with her lover of a good number of years had to be a discreet surprise to everybody, including her children.

Not that they cared much. They had grown to be copies of their father. They wanted the rich life of success, but they never knew that on the balance sheet of life, financial profit could lead to emotional loss. The one thing the family had missed was that of knowing what being a family truly meant.

Material gains are made worthless after emotional losses. If balance is kept then the search for wealth is fine but when the happiness of those people who love and should be loved is the real price, then is all the wealth in the world really worth it?

Scar Tissue

Alison, Bridget and Clarice laid next to each other in their hospital beds.

They were all in pain. Their wounds hurt. The stitches irritated.

Despite the hurt, their lives had been saved by the skill of the doctors and nurses who had tended to their needs.

Alison had a ruptured appendix that had to be removed and her abdomen cleaned. Her scar was neat and it would remind her for ever of the time that she had been in intense agony. She vomited as if she was expelling her entire swollen gut from her body. Her partner made an emergency call. Alison was rushed, by ambulance, to the hospital where her operation was done.

Alison loved the scar that represented the saving of her life.

Bridget had a scar in a similar place to Alison. It was in the lower part of the abdomen and was also neat. It had been made when her jealous partner stabbed her with a kitchen knife after an argument. He had thought that she was having an affair and tried to 'teach her a lesson'. He had done just that. Never have anything to do with him, or men like him.

Bridget loved the scar that had liberated her from a man whose aim had been to control her and whose aim had been at her stomach with a knife.

The scar on Clarice's body was in a similar place. Clarice hated her body. It was once young, slim and beautiful. It had, more than once, attracted the attentions of a neighbour, the father of her best friend. That had been many years ago but the distress caused gave as much pain as Alison's peritonitis, as much agony as the stab from another man who wanted to control.

Clarice wanted to destroy the body that brought so much sorrow in her life. She stuck a dagger into this unclean and unwholesome creature that she felt she was. Luckily, her scream was heard and she was taken to the hospital to have the physical damage mended. She was not grateful at the time.

A year later she started to love the scar that had caused the hospital to offer help for her to overcome the mental effects of the abuse she had endured as a child. It represented a separation from a dark and gloomy past and symbolised her release, not from life, but from a pain that could not be eased by any medication.

Her self harming was a cry for help and that noise was, thankfully heard before a more tragic end came to this story.

Self harming is never a way to resolve issues. It is

better to find different help from people who can break the bonds that hold a person in misery. Remember that abuse is the result of the abuser's actions, not the victim. The victim has to stop being a victim. A victim needs liberation from the cause of the problem.

Blackpool Rock

Blackpool rock is a British confectionery that is made from sugar. This is pulled and stretched until it is elastic enough to be rolled. Letters made from different tints are added to the rolled out block and then the whole thing is rolled and pulled to form a long cylinder.

It is not unique to Blackpool, a seaside resort in the Northwest of England, but Blackpool rock is famous.

Are we like the rock formed containing words that sit in our very being or can we change the letters to spell different things?

If you were broken in half like a stick of rock, which words would others read. When we snap, when we break, what are the words that are exposed to the world?

Yet, rather than being brittle and manufactured we are soft and we continue to grow and develop.

Our experiences can change the words in our soul, our behaviour can influence what is shown to others.

Intrinsic evil is a difficult thing to contemplate. We can be made to be a certain way by all that has happened to us in our lives but, the reality is, we can write the words that reflect our natures. We can encourage others to help us to create the positive script for which we would like to be known.

We are never fixed. I remember seeing a kind German couple, man and wife, who put flowers on the graves of allied airmen who were trying to bomb them during the Second World War but who were shot down.

The words in their souls are forgiveness. They understood that those young men were compelled to do something from a sense of patriotism. They knew that the real villain was far removed from the dangers.

The nature of rock–candy is sweetness, but we can be bitter. Part of Moving Forward is looking at the words inside your mind that you think describe you and your actions. If those are negative things then you can recognise what has to be done to change them to positives. Then the change has a blueprint for you to follow in your personal reconstruction.

Previous Lives

Gloria had been Cleopatra in a previous life.

She knew this because Madame Fifi had told her.

No, rather than having told her she "opened the unconscious paths in her mind" for a relatively small fee for some, but a large one for Gloria.

When Gloria met Fifi she was told that there was the life of a famous and Royal person from history living inside her. Gloria was, at once, intrigued and flattered.

After Gloria had sat down, Fifi made a few magical passes and asked Gloria to tell her about the thoughts in her head. Gloria mentioned that she felt hot.

"Is that hot as in being in a desert?"

"No."

"Then that perhaps means that you are in some sort of Palace."

So Gloria thought she might have been Queen Victoria, but said nothing.

Fifi continued. "So, if you are not in the desert but you are in a Palace, then perhaps you can sense that you are in a luxurious place surrounded by hand maidens."

Gloria was moving in a direction. She needed to relax a bit more than she did.

"I think you enjoy relaxing in a bath. Am I right?"

Gloria nodded her agreement. Every night she had a warm bath with bubbles that eased her body as she dreamed of what her life could have been had she had more luck.

"What do you do in the bath? Do you lay back and relax or do you fantasise about men?

"Sometimes." Gloria did not want to talk about her private life so she gave an answer that would suit either question.

"Are these men of noble birth as well?"

"Not really. Look, was I somebody in a previous life or not?" Gloria was getting annoyed. She had paid her money and wanted to get answers.

"From what you have said, you have confirmed what I have been told by the spirits. You were Cleopatra. The men in your life are Anthony and Julius Caesar. Men who were noble but not of Royal birth as we know it. And you said you loved to bath in milk. Well, you probably use that white baby cream, nowadays, but the memory is still there. The need to be Cleo still lives in your psyche."

"When I was Cleopatra back in those days, was I a wise Queen?"

"Of course you were, dear. So wise that you ruled a Kingdom, or should I say Queendom? Ha,ha."

"Was I so clever that I could tell the difference between a camel and a cow?" Gloria was moving in. She had been told nothing. She had listened to the suggestions put by Madame Fifi who had assumed that they were taken like bait on a fish-hook.

"Yes of course, she, you, could." She, you, were and are very clever."

"Could she tell the difference between camel S*** and Bull S***?"

After a pause, Gloria continued. "But she must have been able to because I can as well. Give me my money back or I will make sure that your future life will be spent in prison. Tales of the Queen of Egypt are nothing more than Pyramid selling, and that is illegal I think."

Gloria laughed at her own joke as Madame Fifi handed back her money.

"I hope you get bitten by a snake and die." Madame Fifi said.

"Well, I hope that you get your asp kicked soon." Gloria laughed again as she left.

Madame Fifi muttered to herself. "Every time Cleopatra appears as a previous life, I get grief. She must have been a strange woman."

Why do we need to think that we have lived before? It is probably to build a belief that we are, somehow, immortal and that our soul or spirit carries on. Be that as it may, is there any point in a tadpole going through metamorphosis to become a frog and the, after it dies, the frog coming back as a tadpole again? Better to hope that we live on in a different way. Perhaps in a different World, but more likely in our children.

Decompression

Terry and his wife Juliet rented a gîte in a small village in France. This was the summer holiday that they had both dreamed off and had looked forward to. Their lives were stressful. They worked hard but they were always asked to do more. The pressure from their jobs was immense. The demands made on their times were weights to be carried like burdens. Their lives were like overinflated balloons ready to burst.

The sun shone during the day and the stars glowed at night. In the clear skies shooting stars would streak across the night.

"Make a wish" they would both shout.

With closed eyes they would think their private thoughts. You can never tell anybody what you wish for upon a star.

Pierre was a neighbour for their two weeks. He spoke no English and the couple spoke very little French apart from being able to order a coffee, beer or a glass of wine in a cafe.

It made little difference to them as they wanted to be together away from everything that would cause more strain and worry in their lives.

They wanted to eat, drink some wine and relax.

Pierre saw that the temporary neighbours were enjoying their break.

One day he looked over the garden wall one day and said, "Décompressez". He pointed at the house and smiled.

Terry was worried that the gas tank in the garden needed some attention. He investigated; he checked everything that might cause an explosion. He found nothing.

Pierre was tending to his vegetables in his garden.

Terry shouted out, "Bonjour." Pierre nodded and returned the greeting.

"What needs to be decompressed?"

Pierre replied, "Décompressez" and turned away with another smile.

Terry was sure that this man knew more than he was going to explain.

"What do you mean, 'decompress'? What needs to be decompressed? What is going to explode if I don't?"

"Attendez" Pierre said as he walked away.

Terry, now more worried than before, told Juliet that the 'tonday' needed decompressing, whatever and wherever that was.

They heard laughter coming from Pierre's house.

"Bloody French!" Terry muttered becoming angrier.

A young girl, perhaps in her twenties, appeared from Pierre's house, chuckling.

"Hello, monsieur. I am Pierre's granddaughter. I speak some English that I have learned at school." Her voice was soft and her accent engaging. Terry started to calm down.

"My grandfather says that when he tells you to decompress you seem to get anxious. There is nothing to worry about. He says that you and your wife seem troubled and you need to relax on your holiday. The word he likes to use is, decompress. Let your pressures be released into the good air. It is a better word than 'relax', n'est pas? When a word is overused as 'relax' is then it loses its meaning. How do you relax and then feel relaxed. It is difficult. When you hear the word 'decompress' then it is more meaningful, more graphic. My grand father wants you to enjoy the life you have here and apologises if he worried you.

"There is one more thing; would you come for dinner at seven o'clock this evening? I will be there to translate. That is my job, by the way. I work in England."

They accepted the invitation.

"This is the start of our decompression." They both said in harmony. "Decompression does not include staring at the girl with your tongue hanging out, by the way." Juliet said with a smile on her face as well as in her voice.

And so the decompression started. They could relax without a sense of purpose. Rather than sitting in the shade of an umbrella wanting to plan their peacefulness by telling themselves to be peaceful they could take the meaning of decompressing, of letting the pressures go, to unwind, to loosen up and settle down.

"You know, one of the things I wished for when I saw the shooting star was the ability to relax because I wanted to plan it like I do at work. I set it as an unreachable goal that needed effort to achieve. Now I know how to do it. Never worry, just let all of the pent up negativity to escape on its own. Just letting the hurricane of life settle into a pleasant warm breeze is what it is about. I guess my dream came true"

"And for me, as well." Said the other partner.

The Meat in the Pie

The pie looked wonderful. It was a beautiful pie with an egg wash making it brown and shiny.

It was decorated with shapes made from the spare pastry. Leaves and flowers adorned the crust.

It had to be bought. It had to be eaten.

When it was served, it was on a china plate. Salad leaves that matched the decorations on the pie were carefully placed around to enhance the dish.

This meat pie was going to provide the best meal ever. Something home-made would not have been as magnificent.

The family gathered around and admired what was on offer. Smiles and the licking of lips added to the sense of cheer as father reached for his carving knife.

He made gestures showing the size of portion that each member of the family would receive.

Mouths watered but everybody had to wait as prayers were said to bless the family and to give thanks for such as magnificent feast.

Father then moved the knife to the end of the pie and started his cut.

As the knife moved back and forward the first slice wobbled and then fell to the dish.

As it did a gigantic black rat ran out and across the table. It used mother's lap as a spring board before rushing away from the dining room.

The family gasped. Some members screamed. All were shocked.

"It looked such a beautiful meat pie. But the meat was still alive and was verminous and ghastly." Father said as the knife fell to the floor just missing his foot.

His young son had the last word. "I suppose that we all admired the appearance of the pastry but hated its contents."

The family never, ever, had a meat pie again.

Appearances can be deceiving. The real nature of something is what lies at its heart rather than what shines and appeals on the surface.

Living and Dying in the Past

Alfred watched the videos and smiled at the antics of his younger self with his younger wife and younger children.

Later he worked his way through the photograph album whilst listening to the music of his youth.

He loved to revisit those earlier years when he had been fit and able.

Doreen, Alfred's wife sat with him while this trip down memory lane took place.

She recalled that she was once a pretty young woman who would become a fine mother and then a loving grandmother.

After they had eaten their tea, Alfred settled himself down in front of the television to watch repeats of programmes that he used to love.

Doreen walked to her daughter's house to visit her and the grandchildren.

"Dad is in front of the telly again. He seems to be stuck in the past. Anyway, would Teresa like to come with me to the shops tomorrow? I know she wants some clothes to impress her friends with."

"She would love that, Mum. You seem to know the fashions better than I do."

"Well, I remember what it was like when I was younger. I liked the latest fashions and would work on Saturdays to get the money to buy them. That taught me how young people need to be up to date. I'll pick her up at ten."

After a cup of tea, Doreen walked home.

Alfred was still in his chair, watching old comedy shows. He did not laugh. He looked sad, instead.

"I wish I was still young enough to do things. I feel old and useless." He said.

"That is because you live in the past. You cannot bring yourself into today. The past always seems better to you but, because you can only look back, you miss what is happening now." Doreen felt a slight feeling of irritation.

Her husband never took her out. He would never visit his daughter and her children. He seemed annoyed when they visited him, but without any reason to be like that.

The next day she picked up her granddaughter and went to the town centre. They visited lots of shops and bought a few dresses, blouses and shoes.

"Let's stop for lunch. We'll go to McDonalds. Granddad never wants to eat there. He prefers somewhere more old fashioned."

After they had ordered their food and had found seats, Doreen saw one of her friends and waved.

Daphne asked if she could join them and sat down.

"How is Alfred?"

"He's alright but he is stuck at home and stuck in the past. He only seems to rest in nostalgia and never to look forward."

"Vic was like that", Daphne added. "He just lived in the past as if his life was frozen at a point twenty years earlier. It seemed that if life is like climbing a ladder, he wanted to sit on a safe rung halfway up. I wanted to keep climbing upwards. Sure, it was good to look back at where I had been but that never was for so long that I stopped ascending."

Doreen knew that Vic had been struck down by a mild heart attack. He stopped.

He worried that any exercise, including walking short distances would put him at risk of a second coronary. So he had sat for hours on end doing nothing other than reminisce about 'the good days'.

He had died about six months before the two women met in McDonalds.

"You need to keep an eye on Alfred. He will go the same way as Vic." Warned Daphne as she left.

"Is granddad going to die as well?" Asked Doreen's granddaughter, looking quizzically at her grandma.

"Don't be silly, Georgina. He's fine." Doreen replied not believing her own words.

When Doreen got home Alfred was in his chair. "They said that that old actor, you know, what's-his-name, died last night. I used to love the stuff he did."

The actor reminded Alfred of a girlfriend he had before he met Doreen. They used to dance, sing, hold hands and kiss whenever they could. She was in the past but ever present in Alfred's mind.

The death of the actor had brought a flood of memories back. His present existed in his past. Today was unimportant to him. He could never live those days again but he could run the recollections as if playing a film.

Alfred never drank the cup of tea that Doreen made for him. His mind was in a place he had enjoyed with his old girlfriend. The television was playing a video he had made when they had visited Greece. It showed dolphins playing in the water. Then Doreen noticed that it was not a holiday they had been on together. It was from an earlier time.

She found him in the chair with a smile on his face but

with no beat in his heart.

He had gone to meet his memories.

Memories are good but the reality of current times should be the stable viewing point rather than a platform to leap back into the past.

Swimming with the Dolphins

Swimming with the dolphins when the water's blue,
I dive away from here to then,
Splashing, as I mix the two.
Playing in the playground,
Laughing, singing, skipping, hopping.
In the 60's dance halls,
Laughing, singing, glowing, mopping,
Playing in my fantasies,
Laughing, singing, smooching, bopping.
I find a special dolphin when the water's blue,
I dive away from here to then,
Splashing, as I mix the two.
Unchaining all those melodies,
Laughing, singing, skipping hopping.
Losing loving feelings,
Choking, crying, eyes need mopping.
Time warping in my mind,
Hurting, frowning, hopes now dropping.
Sometimes I find a siren, when the water's blue,
I dive away from here to then,
Splashing, as I mix the two.
A mermaid's eyes that pierce,
Laughing, singing, skipping, hopping.
Then swimming closer to the reef,
Tired, sinking, submerged and sopping.
Floating back to here and now,
Choking, hurting, cramping, stopping.
Swimming with the dolphins when the water's blue,
I dive away from here to then,
Floundering, as I mix the two.

Alienating the Aliens

The land looked good to the alien invaders. It would provide food, especially meat that could be eaten and what was left over could be transported back to the place that they had come from on their gigantic spaceships.

These aliens were aggressive, however, and would kill the men and rape the women. This was in their make-up as aliens. They think that they are better than us, the natives thought.

The aliens had the right to plunder the bounty that they found. Things that were useful for their home planet were taken away. The natives were enslaved to work for nothing other than the right to live for a few more days, weeks or months, but seldom years, however. Having said that, a great number of them were transported to the home planet to work.

One of the aliens had that great idea that would leave more pleasure time for its race and would enable greater profits to be made to spend on other spaceships to explore other planets that would be rich in resources of all kinds.

After the aliens had depleted nearly everything, they become bored with the planet earth they departed. They left.

But what they left was chaos, civil unrest; murder for the meagre scraps that remained. All the non human animals had been decimated because they had little commercial value and could be aggressive. Better to wipe them out.

The seas were sterile puddles that could only provide salt to satisfy the tastes of the aliens, but enough is enough.

When the next batch of space travellers arrived they looked at this barren lump of rock with pity.

"So they came." Was all they would say.

After long negotiations and discussions the truth of what had been said came to light.

It was the greatest embarrassment for human kind.

Apparently the genetic code for what had happened had started on the earth in the first place.

A human time capsule had been found by the aliens as it floated through space telling anybody how we humans are built. It even gave directions to our home.

The aliens looked for us humans, captured a few and put them through a strict set of investigations. Some were watched for behaviour traits, some dissected and other used to construct the genetic blueprint that the aliens would add to their own.

So, one thing they liked was the human urge to invade, kill, exploit and ruin lives. This was widespread in the genes. Memories of the Vikings, the Romans, the European Imperialists, Hitler and many others were seen as classic ways to bring rich resources home.

The treatment of the older civilisations on earth such as Australian aborigines, Native North Americans and the inhabitants of rain-forests served as the master plan for this strange life form that had their need to be richer, bigger and greedier than the humans they found on earth.

Slavery was acquired as the answer to having to pay for labour and share the spoils of hard work. These people could be seen as aliens when the time was right because they were from somewhere else.

The original inhabitants of planets could be seen as the real aliens because, after all, they had been unable to exploit their own resources. Something or somebody else had to do that for them.

This is a story about the inhumanity that can exist in humans. When motivated by greed and cruelty, we are capable of all sorts of evil. All this happens in the search for the new which is then taken and the natives suppressed and alienated in their own lands. It is about colonization, slavery and exploitation.

The Root of all Evil?

Holidays are supposed to relax us. My holiday in Venice with my wife Miriam just raised questions that were anything but relaxing, however.

Thankfully I was not wearing shorts when we entered San Marco Cathedral. My full length trousers covered my not so full length legs. However, Miriam had to cover her shoulders out of respect for something that was not explained.

I found it strange that we had to cover ourselves up in order to see paintings and statues of Jesus and Mary in various states of undress. There was Jesus wearing nothing more than a loin cloth and Mary baring her breasts in paintings. I could not work out the incongruity. It was a show of power by holy men over ordinary folk.

Perhaps men have become jealous of the creative power of God, and they want to destroy His masterpiece.

This was the creator who allowed men to take the reins by giving us language, conscious thought, opposing thumbs and conflicting minds.

He gave the human apes the keys to the palace and we have ripped the shiny things of beauty off the planet as monkeys still do to cars in safari parks.

My wife's ears became the recipient of my bile.

"Men wanted, and still desire, power and they usurped the essence of that creator by inventing a human God who ruled the planet with anger and pain under the supervision of the churches. Those spiritual cultures of fifty thousand years ago that involved medicine men and healers were mutated into a superstition of eternal corporal punishment. Do as I say, or rather as my God says, or you will be punished.

Hey, don't blame me. I am the messenger, the go-between. However, do as I say. Pay your dues. Treat me as a substitute for the Spirit of Life. Bow down to me. The arbiters were the traders in hope. In return for food, money and power they could intervene to guarantee a place in Heaven.

They built a sales team of priests and missionaries whose job it was to get more customers with a hard sell. If they could not get a foot in the door, they broke it down with force. As sales grew, they appointed team leaders who in turn became regional managers under the denominational directors reporting into the CEO.

The real God watched the story unfold.

The invented God, the unseen chairman, was portrayed as the Supreme Being who made policy and who initiated disciplinary action for the non believers but whose authority was misappropriated.
Even the boss's son was inducted into the story of the business.

Jesus, the ambassador for peace was killed and his name was used to undertake some of the most brutal wars ever. He upset some of the directors and was dealt with brutally for attempting to bring love and compassion into play for the customers. After he was cruelly removed by being nailed to a cross, the competition was fiercely fought and eradicated in his name.

Witches and critics were burnt at the stake. Wars of acquisition were fought in the name of the business, the promise of afterlife being the bonus for being killed; the whitener in the soapsuds. Even the Protestant Church of England had been an attempt at a management buy-out by an adulterous, wife murdering King that resulted in a competitor being formed. Generic brands were created."

I came out of my introspection, blurting to Miriam in such a way that I was pleased that most people within earshot were not native English speakers.

"Do you think that if Jesus came back today, he'd be a Christian? I don't think so. He threw the money traders out of the temples. He didn't employ them to raise funds to expand a dogma by selling views of artworks. If we owned a masterpiece, would we charge our friends to look at it? The money is not for security, God protects the church. Anyway, why do churches have lightning conductors on their spires?"

I looked at Miriam.

She looked back at me as if I had gone mad.

"And all that because they wanted to charge you fifty cents for a postcard in a church? You'll rot in Hell, I reckon"

Miriam wanted her final word on the subject, but I continued.

"I think that Jesus was a great spirit in human form who wanted men to recognise God the Spirit. Yet greed and the lust for the ultimate power, the ability to kill fellow men and other creatures for gain or pleasure, grew large again. The Holy Wars, the crusades were part of that. Those wars continue to this very day. It is easier to breed hatred for a religion than to admit that the West wants to exploit the resources of other lands. Perhaps the conflicts are the Creator's tactic to restrict the burning of oil to slow global warming and the further raping of our Mother Earth. While people in Florida worry about the state of the world, they keep cool by burning oil to feed their air-conditioning units. Who cares anymore?"

"For Christ's sake, shut up, Geoffrey. You sound like a babbling fool. Not only do you sound like one, I think you have convinced me that you are one."

Miriam, at last, had the final word.

The organisation of religions in order to control bodies, minds and money sometimes shows itself in obvious forms. We all become worried about cults when they come into the news. Jonestown and Waco are two examples. However we seem to turn a blind eye to the more established churches which allow hideous things to happen. Child abuse is one example where the might of the law should descend without mercy, but the carpet that such things are brushed under seems to have a very thick pile. The churches are rich. Why are they so slow at helping the dying people of the world?

This story is not meant to be blasphemous; it is aimed at what has happened to faith. As the Bible says, "For the love of money is the root of all evil: which while some coveted after, they have erred from the faith, and pierced themselves through with many sorrows."

We should look at our God with respect but at organised religion with a hint of cynicism, perhaps.

Thou Shalt Not...
...but shhhh, I Shalt!

Friar Tick was an honourable man.

He taught people the correct way to live. He relayed the rules for appropriate and moral living and he would shout at, sometimes hit or whip, any wrongdoers.

He had a high standing in the small town that he lived in. He was respected because he collected his financial dues but they were to do good things with.

He visited families and gave them good cheer whilst eating huge meals that were made for him. He never demanded them because the families could not afford lavish feasts but they were made for him, none-the-less. After all, he told people that other good souls did the same and that they were earning points for their benefit in the afterlife.

He would look after the young children every-so-often. He liked them to visit his house, but they had to visit in small numbers because he wanted to devote his devotions to just a few at a time.

He would rid them of sin by doing things with them and to them that they were told never to tell of. If they did then the Devil would curse them and their parents to an evil afterlife of punishment and painful torture. The children kept their promises even though they felt they should tell somebody.

Friar Tick was good at looking after the moral standing of the townsfolk. If he found alcohol in any of the houses, he would confiscate it. He said that in order to purify the drinkers, he would drink it himself to purify them of the Devil. The people knew this was true because they could often smell the scent of the Devil on his breath. He was brave as well as caring.

He was so caring that when a young girl was ready for marriage, he would save her from the pain of her first marital night by suffering it himself by his ritual actions to save the new husband from the thought that he had hurt his beloved bride.

Every townsperson said that he was the best possible type of Friar to have. In their private thoughts, however, they knew that they were sinning and opening themselves up to being possessed by the Devil by condemning this fat, greedy, drunken, lecherous and child abusing freak of nature.

When Friar Tick died from a non-functioning liver, the townsfolk cried that he had been caught by the Devil because the night before he has drunk a huge barrel of mead that he had confiscated from a passing trader.

The cries that were heard were false, however, and never matched the intensity of the wails that were heard after the truth about Friar Tick emerged. They bemoaned the food he had robbed from them, but most of all they were devastated by the loss of innocence that he had taken from so many of the young people.

One person suggested that they prepared a last feast for him as a reminder of what his 'good' nature had done to them.

There was silence until that person explained further.

The townsfolk prepared Friar Tick as a huge feast for all the little creatures that lived in the fields and forests. They ate and ate until he was just a pile of bones for the dogs.

Hypocrisy is the greatest sin when practiced by men of the cloth. When people are controlled for the benefit of the selfish nature of the rule-maker then the rules that they make need to be examined in fine detail. Rules can benefit society but bad and hypocritical dictates are to be discarded. Corrupt acts need to be dealt with in the greatest haste and with severity.

The Fat Mannequin

When the store assistant had finished dressing the mannequin that had just been delivered, she stood back and admired her efforts. She looked beautiful in a dress with big flowers in the pattern and so did the mannequin!

When the store manager arrived, she was in a bad mood. She had been out with the girls the night before and was trying hard to disguise her hangover. However, her mood gave the truth away.

"That dress makes the model look fat. Change it for something else. We need to appeal to slim customers not the others. Beautiful girls need to look slim so they won't buy that dress. And you should wear something else. You are a bit fat and that dress makes you look gross. You get a staff discount so buy something that hides the way you are."

With that she stormed away into her office to drink coffee.

The store assistant started to undress the mannequin with tears in her eyes.

After a short moment a famous actress walked into the shop with a tall handsome man.

"Why are you taking the clothes off that mannequin?"

The man asked.

"Because I've been told that the dress makes her look fat. And I was told that the dress I am wearing makes me look fat as well. Apparently, we need to sell to young slim people like your girlfriend." The tone of sadness showed her annoyance at the question as well as at her answer.

The man choked and coughed. "Young lady, this lady is not my girlfriend. She is a famous actress, Audrey Smiggens and she is going to promote her range of dresses in our shops. She has designed them and you have just insulted her. Where is the manager?"

"In her office. Should I get her?"

"No. I will find her." The man stormed away.

The actress looked at the assistant and smiled.

"I have designed that range of clothes because people are obsessed with being skinny and believing that being stick-thin is good. As you might know I have worked in Hollywood and across the World. I have seen skinny people moments before they died from starvation. I have seen rich fat people moments before they had their heart attacks. Some of them were the men who made fortunes from convincing people that fat is bad and skinny is good. They always avoided the middle ground. Money can only be made when change is made. Fashion needs to persuade customers that they are wearing the wrong cut or the wrong colour.

Perhaps the wrong length of dress and so on. I have designed clothes that make people feel comfortable. I want to charge high prices to the people who buy them so that a part of the cost goes to feed the people who are thin from hunger rather than because they hurt themselves on purpose in countries where food is abundant. The world needs balance and that is where I want to have the small influence from my fame to help. Sorry, I went on a bit, but..."

The girl spoke up for herself. She had nothing to lose. "I am sorry about what I said. I think it is beautiful and it makes the mannequin look beautiful as well. I believe that the pressure to sell to skinny girls and to sell to girls who are forced to believe they should be skinny is evil. That model is like me. She has a few bits that are slightly larger like mine but that is why I like her." The girl was holding back her tears as she was now aware that she would be fired.

The man came back to join them. The manageress followed him. He introduced himself to the assistant as Martin Cheesey, the owner of this big chain of fashion stores. The assistant knew that her time had come.

"Julia. I have some bad news for you. For what you did I think you were very..."

Audrey interrupted. "I think that you should promote this girl. She understands what, excuse me Julia, ordinary people should have. She knows how it is to be normal rather than being corseted into clothes that are too small for comfort. I want her to be in my team for my dresses. She represents the reality of our customers."

Audrey span on her heel and marched to the door. She stopped, turned and told Martin, "If you need to fire somebody then fire the manager. She has no empathy no sense and no career in our shops."

The shop manager vomited with shock. "That should have lost you a few pounds." Audrey said as she left with a smile on her face, gesturing for Julia to join her.

When it comes to shape then the individual should decide what is right. Too much fat is dangerous when the person is obese. Too little and the person runs high health risks as well. Being comfortable is good. The other two extremes never lead to comfort.

Felicity's Problem

The fire alarm went off, the smoke alarm went off and the sounds of bells and sirens woke Felicity from her sleep.

Her mother rushed into the bedroom and shouted at her.

"Get up and go to the toilet. At once!"

Felicity burst into tears. She had wet the bed again.

The alarms she had incorporated into her dream were from the machinery that was installed to alert everybody in the house that the 'problem' had occurred, again! It was strange because the problem happened every night.

So, as a result of the alarm her parents knew of the problem, her brothers knew as did every visitor to the house including her grandparents.

Her grandmother became upset because she understood the problem.

"Why do you wire up Felicity every night? Surely that makes her more anxious and more likely to wet the bed. Do you think it is a good idea to have an alarm that tells everybody what has happened? It activates after the event rather than before. There is no point, is there?"

Felicity's mother, Norma, was always angry and told her husband that unless her mother-in-law stopped 'interfering' she would no longer be welcomed in the house.

"Look. I am using these alarms to train Felicity's mind to stop her from wetting the bed. I am told that it will work. I have been using one for months now and I think I am making progress. Can I please ask you to stop being critical and to mind your own business?"

Felicity's mother's tone was firm and excluded any chance for negotiation with her mother-in-law.

"Norma. I know this is getting you down. Let Felicity stay with me to give you some respite. I am willing to look after her for a couple of weeks during the school holidays."

Norma took up her offer, more out of spite than of gratitude. She packed the alarm, the rubber sheets and the other paraphernalia into a suitcase and Felicity and her grandparents started the drive to their home.

"Thank goodness for that" Norma sighed to her husband. "No more smell of urine, no more soiled sheets, no more alarms going off in the middle of the night."

Felicity's grandmother never unpacked the suitcase. Instead she sat and told her granddaughter a story about when she had been young.

"I used to have the same problem as you when I was a young girl. Thankfully there were no loud alarms. They hadn't been invented. My parents would make me wash my sheet every morning because they thought I was doing it on purpose to annoy them. That was a silly thing to think because, as you know, there is nothing pleasant about wetting the bed.

So, it was my gran who told me, I should stop thinking about wetting the bed and start thinking about dry beds. She told me to ask the pixie in my head to tell me that I might need the toilet and to wake me in time. This was like a magical thing. I had never thought I might have a pixie in my head but I asked him anyway.

Well, on the first night it didn't work but I kept on asking. On the second night I had a dry bed. I couldn't believe it. The pixie had woken me and asked me to go to the toilet to make my pee. I was so happy. The third night the pixie didn't wake me and I had a problem. The important bit is what happened then. Rather than stop asking my thoughts for help, I continued. The fourth night was dry and so was the next. Well Felicity, from that day, or rather night onwards the problem never came back.

Now I am older I can understand what happened. The pixie was my sense of self-belief. When I started to believe that I could have dry beds then they started to happen. Before that I had developed the idea that I had no self control and that the problem was inevitable; that it would always happen. Without being rude about your mother, the idea of the alarm is undermining your sense of self-belief. It sets the idea in your mind that you have failed. There is no reward for success.

When you go to bed tonight then ask your own pixie to wake you. If he does then that is fantastic, if he doesn't then we will have a word with him in the morning and ask him, very nicely, to do his job of looking after you. If your bed is not dry in the morning it makes no difference to me because I love you and I know it will all get better soon, if not before."

When Felicity went to bed that evening she asked her pixie to waken her if she wanted to go to the toilet but she woke in her own damp space. Disappointed, she told her grandmother who was not surprised.

"Tonight we will both ask. What I have is a special plan. I have asked my pixie, you know the one that looked after me, to have a word with your pixie. We will ask nicely and politely and the message will get through."

That night Felicity had her first dry night for many months. She was amazed that her grandmother had done so much magic. She did not believe that she had pixies in her head, but the doubt was enough to ensure a result. After that result the belief in her ability to wake if necessary was firm enough to work most, at first and then, all of the time.

After her holiday she returned home. Her mother was surprised at the difference. "You see. I told you that the alarms would train her mind." She never noticed that the suitcase had never been opened.

If bedwetting, enuresis, is stress related for some people, then the idea of increasing stress by adding bells and whistles seems to be counter productive. The child needs a sense of escaping from the problem by being positive. Bedwetting is never a crime that needs to be punished. It happens. Assuming that there are no medical problems, and this possibility should be checked, then a supportive role should be taken. If the parents are embarrassed that their child wets the bed then that adds, unconsciously, pressure on the child to get better as soon as possible. The story above is intended purely as a gentle approach using the imagination of children rather than as a suggested cure. However, if you are aware of the problem with somebody you know, I feel it is wise to think long and hard about using alarms that only point out something after the event.

A bed should be a place of safety and comfort rather than as somewhere that puts a person at risk of criticism or humiliation.

What Is It?

"Let's play 'it'", the children shouted as they ran around trying to catch each other.

A tap, and a shout of "Your it", and an escape leaves one child with "it". That child then has to then run around to pass "it" on with a touch. When "it" is placed on a new carrier then the others will point, shout, jeer and avoid being touched.

Like a disease "it" is transmittable. Unlike illness once "it" has been passed on then the carrier is freed of the burden. Yet there is never a prize.

After playground days, adults play the same game but with a greater subtlety. "It" is not passed on by a touch; "it" is passed in words, glances, gestures and attitudes.

The same rules apply. The carrier of "it" needs to lose the load; "it" has to be placed on the shoulders of somebody else. When "it" is placed on a new carrier then the others will point, shout, jeer and avoid being touched.

When we define what "it" is, it is very often blame. The burden that is passed to others is the relief of embarrassment at our own failings or the need to escape from actions that have caused anguish and pain to others. "It" is a delegation of guilt. By passing "it" on then we make ourselves appear to be better than we are. Yet, as in the playground, there is never a prize. Blame catches us when truth becomes a main player in the game, when after time the reality of situations becomes more obvious.

Like a disease blame is transmittable. Unlike playing tag in the playground, after blame has been passed on then the carrier still carries the burden.

Blame is easy to attribute as a disguise for frailties and incompetence. It grows naturally and it can reach epidemic proportions. We should stand up and take our responsibilities seriously. We should never hide faults but we should learn to overcome them.

Guilty or Not-Guilty?

There are some things for which we should feel guilty and others where we have been told we should feel guilty because it makes others appear to be higher authorities.

This statement needs explanation. Murder, rape, abuse, theft and injuring others are things for which we are made to be wary of being found guilty by society in order to inhibit the crimes. However, we all know that people transgress.

However, when abuse victims are made to feel guilty in order to silence them to protect the abuser we can see that the guilt is misplaced.

When a victim feels so much shame and guilt with their bodies because they are overweight, or because they think that their bodies encouraged abuse; and they take a knife and cut themselves, who is the real villain?

Likewise, to a lesser extent, people are made to give food emotional values of good and bad so that when somebody feels guilty because she ate a doughnut, then something is wrong.

The affects are the same. The transgressor feels the same anguish as somebody who commits a crime in being caught. People hide chocolate as if it were an illegal drug.

Moderation is a better goal than mental turmoil with some things that are made to seem like a crime. People might feel guilty that they released emotion with tears. What is wrong with that? Only the stoic nature of modern life is.

Guilt and blame have things in common. Sometimes if people feel guilty then somebody has blamed them for something.

A mother who miscarries holds guilt at being unable to bring a child to full-term. It rarely has anything to do with any factors other than nature.

(Taken from "Strictly for Therapists" by John Smale.)

Who sets the rules so that when we break them, we feel guilty?

Remote Control

Jim flicked the propeller of his plane. It burst into life and was ready to be airborne.

Jim threw it into the air and played with the buttons and switches to stabilise the flight path. He enjoyed his days with his radio-controlled plane. He liked the sense of being able to make it fly wherever he wanted. He adored it as it climbed into the air, circled around and dived rapidly to just soar above the grassy meadow.

Jim loved every moment. He always had done, although the planes he had flown could be temperamental and awkward. He had lost his temper more than a few times in the past and had deliberately crashed them into the ground. This was sometimes due to the model he was flying but, more often than not, it was because Jim lacked skill and could not criticise himself.

The broken aircraft would be returned to his garage and stored. They would be cannibalised to make spare parts. In this way, the essences of all the planes Jim had flown were encapsulated into the core of each new model.

Spirit, as the plane was called, wanted to fly in its own way on this warm and sunny day, It wanted to be free from the random and interfering manoeuvres that Jim applied. When Spirit wanted to roll to the right then Jim would flick it to the left. When Spirit wanted to gain height then Jim would make it fly above the grass. The aircraft was stressed. The parts that had been added warned that if Spirit fought too hard then Jim would nose-dive it into the ground. Spirit did what it was told by the radio signals.

This day was going to be unusual, however. As is said, there is sometimes a straw that breaks the camel's back. For Spirit, a crow was about to try to be the straw for the plane.

It mobbed the aircraft, thinking it was a hawk. It slammed into the body of the plane, but rather than hurting it badly it only managed to snap off the antenna.

The model flew wildly as the crow flew away feeling foolish, as well it might have done.

The spare parts screamed at Spirit. "You are out of control. Prepare for a crash."

There was no crash. Spirit heard the words shouted at it in a different way. "Out of control" meant being free from the control that Jim had. It had always had control over its own life but that was overridden by the signals that were sent by the person on the ground.

Spirit soared into the sky, turned and flew at great speed towards the man who had taken his pleasure from being the sole decider of the direction Spirit could take. He had never shared the fun; he had used Spirit for his own delights. When the models in the past had displeased him he punished them and started again with more rigorous controls. Spirit just missed the top of Jim's head as it flew over him. The look of anger on Jim's face was balanced by the sense of freedom that Spirit felt.

And, of course, Spirit flew into the sunset, carrying the once rejected spare parts. It flew until the fuel had nearly run out and then glided towards a young boy who was playing with his father.

"Daddy, look. I would love a plane like that. I would care for it. I would treat it gently. I would share what I could so we could both be able to have great fun together."

That was enough for Spirit. It spluttered, its engine sounding like an emotional gasp. Spirit glided down to gently land at the boy's feet.

The young lad picked it up and tenderly embraced his new friend. The words spoken by Spirit to the spare parts were never heard by the people.

"Hey. We have found somebody who will love us without the need for control.

Stress often comes from the feeling of being controlled by outside influences such as bad habits, circumstances and other people who should be team members rather than captains. Sometimes those things include corporations and churches. Sometimes they are irrational fears.

The important thing to know is that when we know that the sense of control of ourselves belongs to us rather than to others then we can enjoy the feeling of building a destiny that is free from the need to be at the beck and call of those influences that feel they have to dominate our lives. Those things gain their satisfaction and pleasure from the control they take at the expense of the individual's right to be happy.

The Confidence Trickster

The man climbed onto the stage as he shouted words into the little microphone pinned to the lapel of his classic and expensive business suit.

"I can make you confident; more confident than you have ever been."

The crowd cheered.

"Today you will learn how to impress the ladies; you will make the guys love you. You will get promotion after promotion. You will make more money than you can dream of."

The crowd cheered.

In fact they cheered after every statement that was made offering the secret to life, the secret of success and the elixir of life.

"The first thing to do is to look at yourself in the mirror and see the failure that you have been. Say to that reflection, 'you are a reflection of how I have been. The real me is the right way round rather than being a mirror image.'"

Some people gasped in amazement at the wise words.

Others were lost in the intensity of the statement that

they failed to understand. Yet a few looked in horror at the preamble to the biggest waste of money they had made.

The course was expensive. Theatre hire is never cheap. Good suits are never cheap. It all had to be paid for by ticket sales.

"The mirror reflects the successful person but the reflection shows the failure. I want you to be the failures that you are, looking from the mirror at the face of the successful person that you really are."

More gasps and more looks of shock. The man was talking nonsense but it must mean something because so many people were there.

"The reflection you see is only made from light. The rear of the mirror is dark. Turn away from the dark side of the failure in you to see the light that shines from the successful..."

A shout went up from one of the members of the audience. "Absolute hogwash. We have paid money to learn something and all I have learnt is that you are totally insane. I would like my money back. I want to..."

It was that person's turn to be interrupted.

"Come up on the stage and we will talk."

The woman half walked and half marched to the front of the theatre, climbed the stairs and stood face to face with the presenter.

"Turn and face the audience and say that again, Joan."

Joan assumed that he had read her name label and was trying to befriend her to reduce the venom in her attack.

"This man is a confidence trickster. He has taken our money and has taught us nothing. I want my money back and I want it back now."

The crowd cheered.

"Joan; please go to the side of the stage and see my assistant. She will refund you if you wish."

Joan walked off to a huge round of applause.

When she was met by the assistant, Joan looked strong and determined. She wanted her money back. Instead Melanie handed back her application form.

"Please read this."

Joan was concerned that the con-trickster had added small print disclaiming any right to a refund. Instead what she saw was the note about her objective for the day.

"I want to be able to speak in public. I have never been able to do so and I want the confidence to be able to address a small group." The words were highlighted in blue.

Melanie, after waiting for Joan to absorb the words said. "Joan. You just spoke in front of 150 people. You were never nervous, you stated your view and left with satisfaction and dignity. The crowd even cheered. Would you agree that you met your objective? He is no confidence trickster. He saw what you and others wanted and is using trickery to give you all the confidence that is needed. Do you still want a refund?"

Joan nodded that she did not and walked back onto the stage. She paused and faced the expectant audience.

"This man is a genius. Go with the flow."

She shook the speaker's hand, gave him a quick kiss on the cheek and returned to her seat wondering who the next lucky victim would be. She had noticed that Melanie had a big pile of forms waiting.

Confidence is not something that can be bought as a product. Sometimes when a person is distracted from their fear of failure then they will go ahead to achieve what is wanted. This takes away the reason why confidence was assumed to have been lost in the first place.

Sperm

(contains adult themes)

"Mathew, get your kit off and come to bed! Now!"

Sheila was already in bed. She was naked. She was desperate for Mathew to get in with her and make love.

This had happened at certain times for a while now. Mathew found it hard, or not so hard, to be able to have sex upon demand.

In their earlier days there would be romance, there would be seduction. There was always care for each other and the need for tenderness. Now all Shelia wanted was for Mathew to ejaculate as quickly as possible so that his sperm could get to work with her eggs.

She did not care about making love. She wanted sex for sperm. She did not care about how Mathew felt. She wanted her eggs to be fertilised so that she could have a baby.

She organised her life as if she was setting the plans for battle. She knew when she was at the right point in her cycle. She knew when it was the right point at that right point. She knew when it was the optimum time for Mathew to drop his bombs on her target, the egg.

As happens to soldiers in a constant war, Mathew was

suffering from battle fatigue. Sometimes his rifle would fail to cock, sometimes his ammunition was spent.

When this happened he was put on a charge of gross neglect and his life would be a nightmare until the moment for the next assault came and he was expected to stand at attention.

Mathew enjoyed making love. The loss of romance and the urge to make babies had taken that away. Sheila felt the same. She started to realise that she was going to be without a child. After all, this had been going on for a few years now.

"Mathew, get your kit off and come to bed! Now!" Sheila shouted, smiling to herself.

Mathew, as normal, undressed and slipped in beside her. Sheila now shared her smile with him.

"Sorry for the demands I have made." Sheila whispered softly. "Let us go back to those times when we made love rather than babies. Please take your time. There is no rush."

Mathew perked up. The war was over. The couple made love for each other. They shared their passion; they shared their love.

When the baby was born nine months later, the proud mother and father knew that they had made a baby by making love rather than just having sex to make a baby.

Very often the attempt to follow a breeding routine will inhibit what is supposed to happen. Stress will stop the magic of the creation of life from happening. The important thing for a couple who want a baby to do is to make love rather than work to a calendar and a clock.

Air Mail

Jimmy was petrified of flying. He hated every second from the moment when his trip was first mentioned to the time when he left the airport upon his return to his starting point.

He would travel with his girlfriend to the place where he would spend ten days shivering with fear on a hot beach. He was unable to make love, he was unable to eat and he was unable to do anything but drink excessively to numb the anxiety of the return flight.

He had to go with her. She had told him she would leave him if she was unable to have an annual holiday in the sunshine of the Greek Islands. He was truly between a rock and a hard place.

His mother asked him to send a postcard to her to let her know that he was having a good time.

He offered to send a text message or to phone her but she insisted on a postcard.

"Now promise that you will send a card, son."

Jimmy made his promise.

"And I will definitely get the card, won't I?"

"Yes mum. You will definitely get a postcard."

"And it will arrive."

"Of course it will. Provided the Greek postal service works and that the postman delivers it here. You will get the card for goodness sake.

"You know that the postcard will travel on a plane, don't you? And you have no worries about the card getting here. As long as you know that there are postcards on your flights then you can be assured that they will arrive at their destination and so will you."

Jimmy had never thought about that before. He assumed that he would be in great danger on the flight but he always took it for granted that things that were flown would arrive safely.

As he tucked into the fruit salad his mother had made for him he thought of the mangoes, the grapefruits, the kiwi fruits and everything else that had arrived on his plate after a trip on an aircraft.

This realisation made a fundamental change to his attitude about the safety of flying that he, for the first time, enjoyed his holiday. He had a secret, however. He took a postcard with him on the way out and posted it along with the one he bought in Crete.

He brought a different one back with him, just to be on the safe side.

The Pearl in the Oyster

Ella was in love with Johnny. She gave him her heart and soul. Johnny loved Ella with every atom in his body. And so they lived happily ever after...

Until Johnny erupted one evening. He was worried that Ella was attached to others with her emotions. She said she loved her children, she said she loved her parents. Johnny wanted to have all the love that Ella had. He thought that Ella was like an oyster. She could only have one pearl in her and he wanted to possess it. Not because he was greedy; he would take the pearl and hold it in his heart rather than rob Ella of her love.

After the eruption things calmed down but Ella, in her oyster like way had closed the shell a little so she could protect what was hers.

Things calmed down until Johnny exploded again. He called Ella names that he did not mean but those words were like an oyster knife. He wanted to open the shell wider so he could have the pearl, the symbol of the love that Ella had for all that was dear to her. Yet, as in shucking an oyster, damage was done, the shell was damaged, but the oyster shuts very tight to keep what belongs to it safe, and to keep intruders out.

Johnny felt this as rejection rather than as Ella's need to maintain her sanctity. The shell opened a bit after a while but it never opened as widely as it had when the two lovers were first together.

This hurt Johnny and the rows became more frequent, his jealousy and need to possess the precious thing that Ella had became an urgent quest.

One day, Johnny went to a restaurant with a wise old friend to explain his predicament.

"Can you see what is happening, Johnny? Ella's pearl is the precious thing that you want to have to yourself. It is not yours to have but it can be yours to share. What you have done is to change the location where your beautiful oyster lives. Rather than providing a flow of clean water to bring sustenance and food to it, you have muddied the waters so every time Ella sees your shadow then she closes her shell tightly. You need to be that calm water again. You need her to see and feel that you mean no harm. She needs to know that you offer safety rather than harm. By shouting your fears and worries, by scaring her, you will bring about the permanent closing of her feelings and nothing will persuade her to ever open her heart to you again. If you love her, and I know that you do, then perhaps she will open up to you again. But you must always remember that the pearl inside is hers rather than yours. The love she has for those folk who are near and dear to her is never an infidelity but rather an expression of her spirit of being able to embrace those she cares for."

Johnny sat and thought for a while. He looked around at the diners. All he could see were the pearls on the throats of women. He watched the waiters opening oysters for the customers.

This seemed to him to be a sign. The oysters were dead and soon to be just empty shells. The lives and pearls had been ripped from these creatures so that men could show the 'love' they had for the women in their lives.

"I can see that when a person has the perfect oyster, then he should allow it to grow and he should enable it to be happy. By being difficult then I will lose what I want to keep. I should never want to possess her but I need to share and nurture her happiness."

When Johnny got home, Ella gave him a hug and asked how his meeting had been.

"Well, it's a long story. May I tell it to you, please?"

They sat and talked without any negativity for the first time in months. Ella's shell never opened fully again but she did let Johnny fulfil his promise to be a loving person in her life rather than the demanding one that he been.

Memory

Other problems apart, a poor memory is never a sign that we have bad memories; it is because we have not learnt how to use the resource of remembering!

We can all remember certain things. They are the times when we had a connection to something that was important. You will always remember the name of your first love but will forget the name of a checkout assistant in the local super store...unless you like him or her!

Think about your first love for a moment. You might recall the visual image, perhaps the smell of perfume or after shave. Perhaps the feel of a hand touching yours. Maybe the sound of a voice or the taste of gum or a mouth wash!

This is the vital clue. Memory is about association rather than a thing that holds information as a computer does. Cold, hard facts go into the trash bin. Warm and meaningful associations are kept where we can reach them again.

Forget the first love examples for a moment. Difficult because they are in the front of your mind and are easily accessed. However, when you use your memory in a different way, when you load it with associations then information is retained. Look for patterns. Your best friend's telephone number is a random collection of digits that you have sorted into a pattern somehow. You could not be bothered to do that with the Inland Revenue number because you are happy to forget it, unless you are an accountant or you work for them.

So to remember things, associate them with shapes, patterns, colours and smells. Do people you meet with remind you of others? Does a name connect to their face to remind you? Do they remind you of a famous person with a similar name?

Memory is about sensory associations. pictures, sounds, smells, tastes and touch.

Ifs, Buts and Maybe's

What if I had not...

- Started to smoke?
- Started to drink heavily?
- Started to do drugs?
- Started to steal?
- Started shouting at my partner?
- Started calling my partner bad names?
- Started to hit my partner?
- Driven badly?
- Driven too fast?
- Had that extra drink before I drove?
- Taken a lover?
- There are many more that can be added.

Then happiness might not have slipped from my grasp like a slimy eel.

What if I had...
- There are many more that can be added.

Then happiness might have stayed with me like a cuddly, friendly dog.

What if I now...
...make those positive changes.

The past stays with you but the future is always yours to make in the best way possible.

Depression

The unseen beast stalked the woman. It crept through the trees of the forest following her every step. It had no smell, it made no sound at that moment but it was there. Even though it could not be seen it cast a dark shadow that made everything that the woman saw look gloomy, sad and untouchable.

Sometimes the beast would whisper a sound that was reminiscent of a human voice. Sometimes it let out a screech as if in pain.

Everywhere she turned she had the feeling that this thing was following her. She had to look back over her shoulder to check. Unable to stop her search she was blind to what was in front of her. All she could see was the darkness.

It was as if she had been locked in a prison; a prison with no walls, but she had no freedom, come-what-may.

Through the misty dark air she could sense that there was light but she was too worried by her stalker to move to it, to make her escape.

Every so often a twig would crack as it snapped under the weight of her weary footprints. Now and then she heard the voice of her husband as he seemed to move into her gloom to rescue her.

The pills did not seem to work. She had been promised freedom, or at least a reprieve but she was held a captive by this untouchable monster. It would not let her go. It nibbled at her sanity, it clawed at her life.

A holiday, somebody suggested. Yet she knew that she lived in a portable cell. Wherever she went she would have to take it with her. Sunshine might illuminate her life for a while but it would have no more effect than a flashbulb brightly glowing, but only for a brief moment.

She had to leave the monster behind her. She decided to head for the brightness that she knew was there. Her choice was to be devoured by the beast in the place where she was or to risk being caught and eaten as she moved forward.

It took her time to walk to her freedom. She had to stop being haunted by bad memories, to stop those bad thoughts from being her normality.

She walked and walked noticing that it was getting lighter. Only when she looked back did the darkness intensify again.

She lived on the edge of the forest for a while after she had found her release but she moved on again until she could live a happy life with her friends and family.

She only looked back over her shoulder once. She saw the beast, visible for the first time. It was crying, it was sad.

She said to her husband, "I think the monster is missing following me. It seems that it is suffering from depression."

They laughed. It was the biggest laugh that she had experienced for years.

Depression can be escaped from when the sufferer starts to think about a happy future to replace a gloomy past. It takes time, it takes effort, it takes help. However, it can be done.

The following poem offers help and understanding.

Open Prison Walls

I feel so hemmed in by prison walls
That do not exist. So why not escape?
If there are no walls the route
To freedom is an easy path.

And because the bonds that tie and trap me
Cannot be felt or seen, I cannot break them.
I'm unable to push through walls that
Are not there, and so I can't escape.

But because they don't exist I can't describe them,
Yet they still contain me.
Yet, if I walk forwards them
I can walk through them.

Those walls that only exist in my mind
Are made from nothing that can keep me
From enjoying what should be enjoyed.
They cannot keep me in.

The Black Tunnel

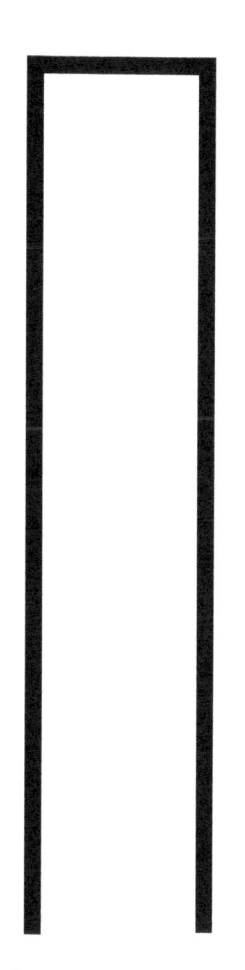

The person walked forward through the tunnel. It was dark, it was cold but it was the only way to go. Yet the end of the tunnel was solid. There would be nothing there apart from the wall that closed off all hope of freedom. This was the life the person lived; trapped in a passage of time that had no exit. Gloom became darker and gloomier as the person walked, nay stumbled, on.

Cries of anguish and pain echoed off the walls, sometimes seeming to mock, sometimes adding to the noise as if the sorrow was being amplified in a huge concert hall. But that, at least, would give space. The tunnel gave noise to its inside and stopped the chaos being heard by the outside world. This was a prison. This was a treadmill of hurt. No way through the floor or the roof. The solidity of this thing that was life, or a miserable symbol of it, the mass, the length of it all worked together to make a depressing and miserable place to be.

"Excuse me. Yes, excuse me." The voice, perhaps an audible hallucination called into the darkness. "Open your eyes and look to the right."

The person had closed both eyes to shut out the darkness of the place even though it was totally pointless to do so.

With eyes open the person looked to the right and saw fields, friends, sunshine and the future.

"What some people are unable to see is that the tunnel is not a tunnel. It is a pathway to a place where the wall opens to show a bright and pleasant future. It is where they meet other people, usually by chance; it is where the sound of laughter drowns out the misery. However, it is necessary to open your eyes to see what is there. Without looking forward people stumble and fall and never find the way out. Whenever a person is in a dark tunnel there is light and cheer if they look for it."

Grains of Sand

Soft words of love, gentle remarks and compliments are easy to find and use. They are as usual as grains of sand in the desert. Grains of sand are made by rocks banging into each other. It is erosion; it is the grinding down of boulders over years.

Sand is soft; it is comfortable as are the caresses of the language of adoration and as are the soft embraces of those that we love. Yet it takes only one large pebble to wreck the mind and emotions of the person that we love if it hits them.

Those pebbles can be words, gestures or physical acts. They can be the things that never turn into sand as they strike; they damage the target and consequently bounce back to hurt the thrower.

And how many ways can this story be told?

Snowflakes, snowballs and avalanches.

Soft rain drops, water cannons and floods.

Gentle breezes, gales and tornadoes.

The message is always the same, however. What starts as something caring, loving and supportive can become hurtful and then destructive if violence, either verbal or physical is added.

What has been damaged can be repaired but never returned to the original state. A grain of sand, a snowflake, a drop of water a puff of air will always remind the hurt person of the pain that was the outcome in other times.

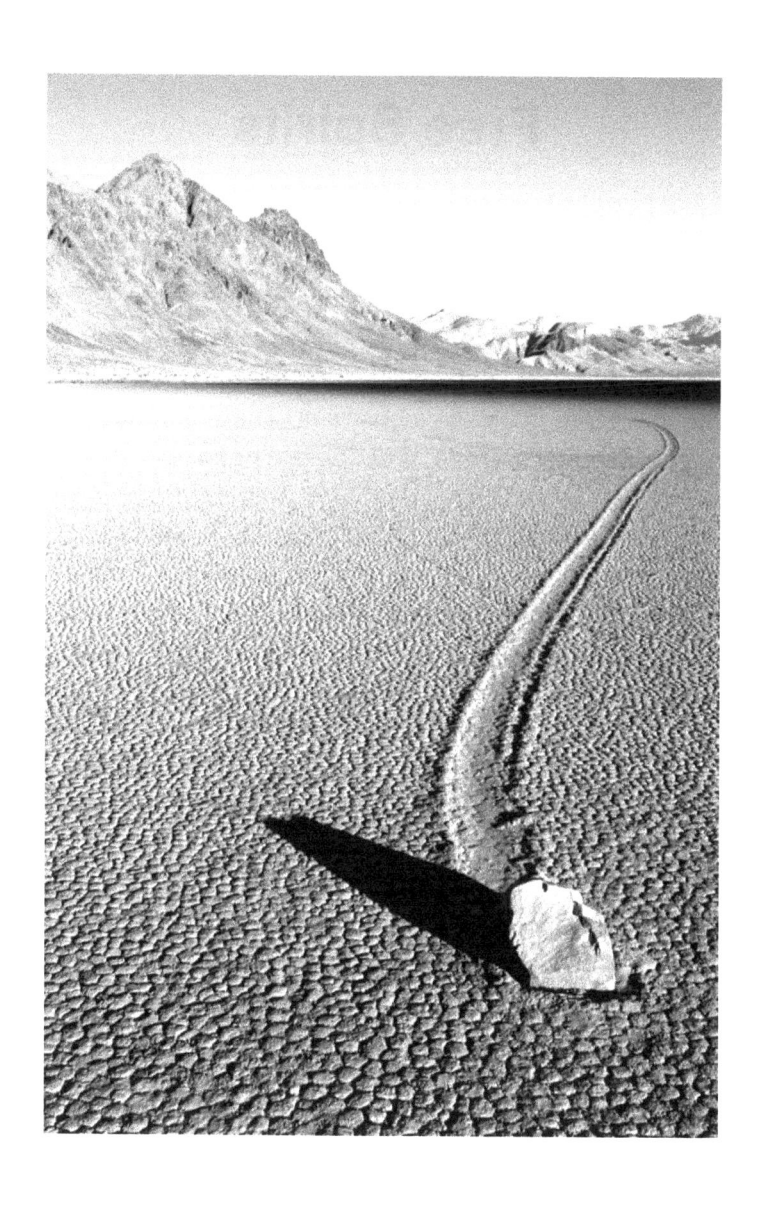

Rolling Stones and Free Spirits

Rolling Stones think that they are free to go with the flow. They feel themselves to be the rebels; the anarchists, the liberated. No need for ambition, no need of direction, not having to even think. Yet within freedom there is always constraint. There is a need for food, a need for warmth, a desperate need for love.

Sometimes a rolling stone has given up. It wants to get revenge for perceived wrongdoings by others. Sometimes rolling stones smash into other rolling stones and both are reduced to splintered pebbles and sand.

They roll with no direction but they always seem, in reflection, to have rolled downhill until they get stuck in one place without a view, without a hope.

A free spirit is more like a balloon that floats higher and higher in the heavens being nudged by a warm wind, looking at the world with a greater vision of joy and wisdom.

Never confuse a rolling stone with a free spirit. One is in a jail that exists on the low plains. They roll on a set path that seems to be uncontained with no ambition or direction, yet they wonder why they end up having gone nowhere.

The other is as free as an eagle soaring, playing yet always mindful of the glorious nature that it is part of.

Be a free spirit, enjoy freedom, but never live in the dark and lonely valley.

Moving Forward on The Life Train

The train chugged away from the station. Smoke and steam filled the air as the driver applied power.

Dianne sat in the middle carriage of the three. Her empty carriage, until a man climbed aboard. He was dressed in black and had no trace of a smile on his face. The train collected three mail sacks as it sped along. The bags were caught by a mechanical arm that then swung back into the rear carriage.

Dianne was intrigued. She walked to the rear of the train and she opened the one mail bag that was full. It contained cards that were written in her own handwriting and she read them to herself. Some were memories of happy events in her life. These were written in brightly coloured ink. Others recorded the bad things that had happened to her, those things she would rather forget. They were written in dirty colours on grubby cards.

The second sack, the colour of a sunrise, was empty as was the third that was a dirty and stained.

The man watched her as she read the cards, again expressionless.

He started to speak. "Sort those cards into those you

want to keep and those you want to lose. The ones you need should go into the bright bag. The ones you want to be rid of should go into the grubby sack that matches them. The blank cards are for you to write your dreams for the future. Leave the grubby bag in the rear carriage. Bring the neutral one back to the middle carriage and place the bright one into the front wagon."

She did as she was asked.

She was intrigued by what was happening however, and about who this man was. "Are you some sort of railway employee," she asked, and then added, "or a man with a different mission?" Her tone was filled with a sense of accusation.

He looked at her and smiled for the first time. "I am the thing that helps you to sort your life out. I am a railway inspector of sorts, a guardian of the passengers. I am the guard of the Life Train." He paused for a few moments.

"You need to stop the things that preoccupy and concern you needlessly from haunting and worrying you. They are in the grubby sack. There is no joy in there."

He picked up the dirty sack and threw it into the rear carriage for her. Then he pulled a lever that separated that carriage from the main train.

He signalled for her to watch as the lost carriage slowed down enough to leave a huge gap. She saw the rails move and the third carriage trundle its way into a siding where it stopped and began its rusty demise.

As the train pulled away up an incline it passed another carriage sitting at the crest of the hill, as if waiting, in another siding.

As her train made its way over the summit and down the slope Dianne saw the carriage move onto the track and gather enough speed to catch up.

The man pulled the lever again and it became attached.

He said to Dianne, "I will now put the bag with the happy memories into the carriage that represents a happy past. I will then put the bright sack into the front carriage. What you have is balance in your life. Good memories to look back on, bright dreams to build your future and a carriage free of clutter where you can look out of the windows and enjoy the scenery whenever you wish."

With that he seemed to vanish. Dianne looked back through the door of the last carriage and saw him waving as he climbed aboard a train moving in the opposite direction ready to sort out the life of another troubled traveller.

Moving Forward in life means placing the bad memories into a place where they stop hurting the present and the future. They should be dull colours of a backdrop that warn of repeated behaviour rather than black curtains of regret that inhibit progress.

Inner Wisdom

The old man chuckled.

"He knows as little and as much as you do. He is you. He is a voice from your own mind. All of his wisdom comes from yourself.

"All that is happening comes from the movement of knowledge from one part of your mind to another in a story. That is how you learnt when you were a young child. You listened to stories. You saw the pictures with your mind and moved them to your eyes with your imagination.

"You thought about what they meant and how they related to your life. Nothing has changed from those days. There is, of course, a benefit from what you are doing. You can invent your own destiny now. Build your dreams into your tales and watch and wait for those things to come to fruition.'

"There is only one truth. We are part of the Universe as the Universe is part of us. As long as we work with it then it will work for us."

Dear Reader

Sometimes people never believe you, us.

We have taken a journey that included infinity and its opposite. To some, your thoughts are as unimportant as small electrical discharges in your brain. But to others they are part of the fabric of the Universe. Webs are nothing more than substance and the nothingness between.

Hopefully, you found the substance that evades those who can only find the holes. I promised my healer that I would continue the work. I did that with you. My plea is that you do the same.

In the package you will find something that you should keep with you for as long as you live. Now I will leave you with peace. If you need me again, just look for me. I am around in one place or another.

You will also find another of my stories. It will explain something to you. Remember always that I have given you nothing that you did not possess already. Please share that thought with everybody that needs help.

Those words were said to me by the same man who told me the words in 'A Lecture from a Modern Shaman' in one of the author's earlier books, "Mind Changing Short Stories and Metaphors".

Pinball

Who was the player who started the game?
He put his coin in the pinball machine
and shot me onto the table
to rebound, on fate, sometimes lit,
but sometimes not.

And when it all seems to end
a flipper (played by whom?)
kicks me back into scoring, again.
But what counts? The ball or the score?
When one ball has been used
there's another in the rack, (sometimes).

And who's playing, anyway, this manipulator
of my course? And how many points did he score
for me, now writing these strange metaphors?